Diagnosing and Treating

Medicus Incomprehensibilis

Diagnosing and Treating *Medicus Incomprehensibilis*

Case Studies in Revising Medical Writing

OSCAR LINARES, MD

DAVID T. DALY

GERTRUDE A. DALY

OXFORD
UNIVERSITY PRESS

OXFORD
UNIVERSITY PRESS

Oxford University Press is a department of the University of Oxford. It furthers
the University's objective of excellence in research, scholarship, and education
by publishing worldwide. Oxford is a registered trade mark of Oxford University
Press in the UK and certain other countries.

Published in the United States of America by Oxford University Press
198 Madison Avenue, New York, NY 10016, United States of America.

Library of Congress Cataloging-in-Publication Data
Names: Linares, Oscar, 1957– author. | Daly, David, 1959– author. | Daly, Gertrude,
1993– author. | Supplement to (work): Linares, Oscar, 1957– Plain English for doctors
and other medical scientists.
Title: Diagnosing and treating medicus incomprehensibilis : case studies in revising medical
writing / Oscar Linares, David T. Daly, Gertrude A. Daly.
Description: Oxford ; New York : Oxford University Press, 2019. | Supplement to Plain English
for doctors and other medical scientists / Oscar Linares, David Daly, Gertrude Daly. 2017. |
Includes bibliographical references and index.
Identifiers: LCCN 2018023984 | ISBN 9780190868680 (pbk. : alk. paper)
Subjects: | MESH: Medical Writing | Terminology as Topic | Case Reports |
Problems and Exercises
Classification: LCC R119 | NLM WZ 18.2 | DDC 808.06/661—dc23
LC record available at https://lccn.loc.gov/2018023984

9 8 7 6 5 4 3 2 1
Printed by WebCom, Inc., Canada

We dedicate this book to the doctors and other medical scientists who write. They strive to make the world a better place by writing about new ways to understand, prevent, treat and cure disease.

CONTENTS

PREFACE

Plain language: communication your audience understands the first time. —Centers for Disease Control and Prevention (USA)[i]

This book presents case studies on revising medical writing in plain English using the methods from our earlier book, *Plain English for Doctors and Other Medical Scientists*.[ii] Each case study looks at a medical journal excerpt and considers, *What makes it hard to read?* and, *How could it be improved to make it clearer and easier to read?*

We designed this book as a rigorous course of study to help you master your skills in plain-English medical science writing. We intend it for anyone who has read *Plain English for Doctors* and would like more practice. You can use it for self-study or as part of a seminar or class.

Why is this book needed? In *Plain English for Doctors,* we described several writing habits that contribute to making medical writing unclear and hard to read. These over-used writing habits are the classic symptoms of *medicus incomprehensibilis*. We gave a tip for treating each symptom. For most exercises, you practiced applying *one* tip, to treat *one* symptom, in *one* short medical journal excerpt. In other words, we gave the diagnosis and you practiced giving the treatment.

In light of this, you may find it hard to apply the same tips to your own writing without someone there to diagnose the symptoms. Revising medical writing into plain English often involves treating several symptoms at the same time. This book can help you meet this challenge, by giving you more practice in diagnosing and treating *medicus incomprehensibilis*.

The book includes 12 case studies based on excerpts from leading peer-reviewed medical journals. The excerpts cover a wide range of medical topics. Each excerpt shows several symptoms of *medicus incomprehensibilis*. Each case study presents questions and gives short exercises, to guide you through the process of diagnosing and treating the symptoms of *medicus incomprehensibilis*.

You write your prescription for revising, make a revision, and compare it to the original. After that, we give our answers to show you how we did these same things.

Good writing takes practice. If you are ready to work towards mastering plain English medical writing, then this book is for you.

Notes

i. Centers for Disease Control and Prevention, "What's Your Point? Put the Most Important Message First," https://www.cdc.gov/healthliteracy/pdf/whatsyourpoint-P.pdf (accessed April 2, 2018).
ii. Oscar Linares, David Daly, and Gertrude Daly, *Plain English for Doctors and Other Medical Scientists* (New York: Oxford University Press, 2017).

ACKNOWLEDGMENTS

We thank and acknowledge several people for their contributions:

Annemarie L. Daly, MD, JD, FACP, for her support and encouragement during the time we wrote this book.

Miriam S. Daly, MD, for her help in reviewing and commenting on the manuscript.

Andrea Knobloch, Allison Pratt, Emily Perry, Jerri Hurlbutt, Virginia Ling, and the other wonderful editors and staff at Oxford University Press who helped bring this book to print.

INTRODUCTION

The most powerful language is also the simplest. When each word has a clear meaning and purpose, readers can move easily through a text and focus on its message. Unfortunately, much writing today is needlessly bureaucratic and difficult to read. —Editors Canada[i]

This book presents 12 case studies on revising medical writing into plain English. It is a companion workbook to our earlier book, *Plain English for Doctors and Other Medical Scientists.*[ii] We wrote this new workbook for anyone who has read *Plain English for Doctors* and would like more practice diagnosing and treating *medicus incomprehensibilis*. It presents a series of challenges in analyzing and revising medical writing to help you master your plain English skills.

What are the case studies like?

Each case study starts by presenting an excerpt from an article published in a leading medical journal, either *The American Journal of Medicine*, *The BMJ (British Medical Journal)*, *JAMA (The Journal of the American Medical Association)*, *JAMA Internal Medicine*, *The Lancet*, *Mayo Clinic Proceedings*, or *The New England Journal of Medicine*. We chose these journals since they contain some of today's best medical science writing and reach a worldwide audience.

Each case study asks questions and gives exercises that focus on *Reading Ease*, *Vivid Language*, and *Logical Reasoning*, the three concepts from *Plain English for Doctors*. These questions guide you through the process of diagnosing symptoms of *medicus incomprehensibilis*, and exploring treatment options. Once you answer the questions, you write your prescription, telling how you would revise the excerpt. Then, you prepare a revision to treat the symptoms and analyze it. At the end, we show our answers, prescription, revision and analysis.

What do you need to know before you start?

Before you start, make sure you're prepared. This means: you've read *Plain English for Doctors* and done the exercises. You've also reviewed the glossary to brush up on key terms.

Excerpts taken out of context

The limits of time and space require that we take each excerpt out of the context of the original article. Don't ever feel you need to look up the original article to get more context. Do look up any word you don't know in a medical dictionary or other reference. Make reasonable assumptions about the context, and revise as best you can.

No criticism

Our goal for this book is to help you master plain English revising skills. Please don't take the fact we chose any excerpt as a criticism of the author or journal. To the contrary, our main goal in choosing articles was to find a set of interesting medical topics. The symptoms of *medicus incomprehensibilis* are so common you can find them almost anywhere.

Somebody might say, one of our revisions *isn't entirely correct, changes the meaning or sense of the original, over-simplifies something,* or *loses some essential scientific content.* Despite our best efforts, we know this may be so. If a revision doesn't involve the original author, it's hard to be sure whether it is correct or captures the sense of the original.

Each revision reflects what we understood of the excerpt taken out of context. But, in some cases, we weren't sure what the excerpt was trying to say, even after careful study. In light of this, we don't claim any revision is the best possible, or better than the original. We had two doctors look at each revision, but this is not the same as peer review.

If we made any mistake in a revision, or if anybody interprets a passage in a different way, perhaps the original wasn't clear. In any event, mistaking meaning or losing key content is never a problem when an author revises their own work. Our goal is to teach you to revise your own work, not to *translate* other people's work.[iii]

Your ideas and judgment may be as good as ours, or better

Each case study asks several different types of questions. Some have just one right answer (e.g., *Are the subject and verb close together in the first 7 or 8 words?*). Others are open-ended or ask for your judgment or creativity (e.g., *What are your first thoughts? What are some shorter words that mean about the same thing?*). For questions like these, we don't expect your answers to always match ours. Your ideas and judgment may be as good as ours, or better.

You may find some questions hard to answer. We certainly did! In writing this book, we discussed each question, answer and revision—often debating among ourselves and, sometimes, changing our minds more than once.

Choices add up

Plain English medical writing involves presenting the right content, clearly and concisely. Writing an article involves making thousands of choices. Some may seem trivial. But these choices add up, either to plain English, *medicus incomprehensibilis*, or something in between. If you make each choice, properly keeping in mind its effect on reading ease and clarity, your choices will always add up to plain English. If the result is not clear and easy to read, you may need to go back and try again.

Trust us to guide you through these case studies. We want you to learn to thoroughly analyze a text, and consider options, before you start to revise. That way, it will become second nature for you to diagnose and treat *medicus incomprehensibilis*. Your writing will become consistently clear and concise, not just *good enough*.

You might find yourself tempted to cut corners—to skip the analysis and just start revising. You can learn something from this; but, if you make a half-hearted effort, you will only get part of the benefit.

WSEG scores

In *Plain English for Doctors*, Concept 1, we presented the WSEG score as a tool to help you diagnose and treat *medicus incomprehensibilis*. We use WSEG scores throughout this book. As a reminder, WSEG is an acronym for:

w—Number of **W**ords
s—Average **S**entence length
E—Flesch reading **E**ase score
G—Flesch-Kincaid **G**rade level

Each case study gives the WSEG score just after the original excerpt, stated in the form (WSEG = *82/27.3/12.9/18.2*). Sometimes, when we compare WSEG scores, we present them in a table.

What *WSEG* scores should you try to achieve?

- Number of words *(W)*—no recommendation, since this depends on many factors.
- Average sentence length *(S)*—Keep sentences 15 words average, 25 words maximum.[iv]
- Reading ease *(E)* and grade level *(G)* scores—Table I-1 gives our recommended ranges of reading ease and grade level scores. Try to get most scores inside the one standard deviation (1 s.d.) range, and all within the two standard deviation (2 s.d.) range.[v]

Table I-1. **Recommended reading ease (*E*) and grade level (*G*) scores**

	Mean	*1 s.d. range*	*2 s.d. range*
Flesch Reading Ease score	57.9	45 to 70	33 to 83
Flesch-Kincaid Grade Level	8.6	6 to 11	4 to 13

How we count words

We sometimes ask you to count the number of words in a sentence. We count words using our computer's spell checker, or by hand, using the same rules. It counts a hyphenated compound (e.g., *resource-limited*) as one word, an open compound (e.g., *student nurse*) as two words, a numeral (e.g., *24.3*) as one word, and an abbreviation or acronym (e.g., *CYP2D6*) as one word.

While average sentence length is important, just how you count words is not. Don't spend too much time fretting over a small difference between your word count and ours.

Writing your prescription

We write our prescription in terms of the tips from *Plain English for Doctors*. However, feel free to write your prescription in whatever way works best for you.

Making your revision

You may not feel comfortable revising someone else's work. You may feel you don't understand the topic well enough, or you don't know enough about what comes before or after the excerpt. If you chop up a long sentence, it will change the narrative tone. For all these issues, make assumptions, and revise as best you can. Keep *essential scientific content*, but try to explain things clearly in your own words.

Don't worry about rendering every nuance of the original author's tone or way of saying things. If you think something is redundant, leave it out. If you think the excerpt fails to explain something that would be helpful to the widest reasonable audience, add it. Make your best judgment about what things may be explained elsewhere in the article.

Analyzing your revision

Your first revision will likely be much easier to read than the original. But, as you review it, you will likely see even more ways to improve it. Perhaps, you can shorten a sentence, use a shorter word, use more-vivid language, change a passive sentence into active, or improve the flow of logic. Feel free to make a second or third revision.

Conclusion

We designed these case studies to help you master skills in plain English medical writing. They take time, but they're worth it. The skills you learn now will serve you throughout your career. Above all, we hope you enjoy learning to treat *medicus incomprehensibilis,* and seeing the result in medical prose that is clearer, easier to read, more logical, and more human.

Notes

i. Editors Canada, "Plain Language," www.editors.ca/plain-language (accessed January 3, 2016).
ii. Oscar Linares, David Daly, and Gertrude Daly, *Plain English for Doctors and Other Medical Scientists* (New York: Oxford University Press 2017).
iii. Ibid.,10.
iv. Ibid., chap. 2.
v. Ibid., chap. 7.

CASE STUDY 1

Allowing More People to Take Part in Research Studies

Plain language is grammatically correct language that includes complete sentence structure and accurate word usage. Plain language is not unprofessional writing or a method of "dumbing down" or "talking down" to the reader. —National Institutes of Health (USA)[1]

A. The excerpt

This case study looks at an excerpt from an article published in *Mayo Clinic Proceedings.*[2] Read the excerpt out loud:

> In addition to basic research, as part of the Precision Medicine Initiative to encourage more individuals to participate in research studies, the NIH is working with the Department of Health and Human Services to revise the Common Rule, which is designed to protect research participants, so that more individuals will be eligible to participate in research. (*WSEG = 56/56.0/0.0/27.3*)

Note: *the NIH* stands for *National Institutes of Health.*

B. Analyzing the excerpt

1. Initial thoughts

What are some of your initial thoughts on this excerpt?

2. Looking at the WSEG score

a. How many words long is this excerpt? ____ What is its "average sentence length?" ____ How does this compare with the recommended average sentence length of 15 words?

b. Do you think this excerpt needs to be just one long sentence, or can it be broken up? Why or why not?

c. Does the reading ease score fall between 45 and 70 (the one standard deviation range)? ____; or between 33 and 83 (the two standard deviation range)? ____

d. Does the grade level fall between 6 and 11 (the one standard deviation range)? ____; or between 4 and 13 (the two standard deviation range)? ____

3. Looking at grammar

a. For each sentence in the excerpt, underline the <u>subject</u> and double underline the <u>main verb</u>.

b. Fill in Table 1-1, answering the questions for the excerpt's one sentence.

Table 1-1. **Analyze the grammar of the sentence**

Sentence	Does the main verb contain a form of to be?	Is the sentence active, passive or neither?	Is the subject abstract or concrete?	Are the subject and verb close together in the first 7–8 words?
1st				

c. If the subject is abstract, explain, in your own words, why it is abstract.

4. Prefer the short word

a. Here is a fresh copy of the excerpt. Underline each <u>long word</u>.

> In addition to basic research, as part of the Precision Medicine Initiative to encourage more individuals to participate in research studies, the NIH is working with the Department of

Health and Human Services to revise the Common Rule, which is designed to protect research participants, so that more individuals will be eligible to participate in research.

b. Count the number of <u>long words</u> and compute long words as a percent of total words.

___ long words/56 total words = ___ %.

c. Double underline any <u>long word</u> you consider a <u>proper name</u> or <u>essential scientific term</u>.

d. For each <u>long word</u> you underlined just once (i.e., skip the essential scientific terms), fill in Table 1-2.

Table 1-2. **Finding shorter words**

Long word	Real-world or abstract?	Shorter words that mean about the same thing

e. Look at the long words listed in Table 1-2. Do any of them have the same or a similar meaning?

f. Fill in Table 1-3 by listing each long word that is a nominalization and giving the root verb or adjective.

Table 1-3. **Find the root verb or adjective for each nominalization**

Nominalization	Root verb or adjective

5. Looking at meaning and logic

a. Here is another copy of the excerpt. The excerpt answers several basic questions: *Who? What? Why? How? With whom? What for? What else?* Write the question above the part(s) of the sentence that answers that question.

> In addition to basic research, as part of the Precision Medicine
>
> Initiative to encourage more individuals to participate in
>
> research studies, the NIH is working with the Department of
>
> Health and Human Services to revise the Common Rule, which
>
> is designed to protect research participants, so that more
>
> individuals will be eligible to participate in research.

b. What is the issue or problem this excerpt deals with?

c. With regard to this issue or problem, does the excerpt: describe it? tell why it is important? offer a solution?

d. Does the excerpt frame the issue or problem in real-world terms or abstract terms? Or does it only imply the issue or problem?

C. Prescription for revising

Write your prescription for revising to treat the symptoms of *medicus incomprehensibilis*. List the things you would recommend to help improve reading ease and clarity.

D. Revision

Revise the excerpt to improve reading ease and clarity.

1. Looking at *WSEG* scores

Compute the WSEG score for your revision. Fill in Table 1-4 to show how your revision compares with the original.

Table 1-4. **Comparing WSEG scores**

WSEG		Original	Revised	Change
W	Number of words	56		
S	Average sentence length	56.0		
E	Flesch Reading Ease score	0.0		
G	Flesch-Kincaid Grade Level	27.3		

2. Looking at grammar

Answer the following questions about your revision:

a. Does each sentence put the subject and verb close together within the first 7 or 8 words? If not, tell why it seemed best to do otherwise.

b. Does each sentence use active voice? If not, tell why it seemed best to do otherwise.

c. Does each sentence use a concrete subject? If not, tell why it seemed best to use an abstract subject.

3. Prefer the short word

a. Underline each <u>long word</u>. Count the number of long words and compute long words as a percent of total words. ___ long words/ ___ total words = ___ %. Compare your answer with the percent of long words in the original. (See §B.4.b.)

b. Double underline any <u>long word</u> you consider a <u>proper name</u> or <u>essential scientific term</u>.

Notes

1. National Institutes of Health, "Plain Language at NIH," https://www.nih.gov/institutes-nih/nih-office-director/office-communications-public-liaison/clear-communication/plain-language (accessed January 2, 2018).
2. Marjorie Jenkins and Virginia Miller, "21st Century Women's Health: Refining with Precision," *Mayo Clinic Proc* 91, no. 6 (June 2016): 697.

Allowing More People to Take Part in Research Studies

Every piece of honest writing contains this tacit message: I wrote this because it's important; I want you to read it; I stand behind it.
—Matthew Grieder[1]

A. The excerpt

This case study looks at an excerpt from an article published in *Mayo Clinic Proceedings*. Read the excerpt out loud:

> In addition to basic research, as part of the Precision Medicine Initiative to encourage more individuals to participate in research studies, the NIH is working with the Department of Health and Human Services to revise the Common Rule, which is designed to protect research participants, so that more individuals will be eligible to participate in research. (*WSEG = 56/56.0/0.0/27.3*)

Note: *the NIH* stands for *National Institutes of Health*.

B. Analyzing the excerpt

1. Initial thoughts

What are some of your initial thoughts on this excerpt?
- *This long sentence covers many ideas.*
- *It is hard to identify the main point.*
- *The science content is low.*

2. Looking at the WSEG score

a. How many words long is this excerpt? <u>56</u> What is its "average sentence length"? <u>56.0</u> How does this compare with the recommended average sentence length of 15 words?
It is almost four times the recommended average.

b. Do you think this excerpt needs to be just one long sentence, or can it be broken up? Why or why not?
We could break up this sentence to make shorter sentences. It contains many ideas that would be easier to understand if they weren't strung together in one long sentence.

c. Does the reading ease score fall between 45 and 70 (the one standard deviation range)? <u>No</u>; or between 33 and 83 (the two standard deviation range)? <u>No</u>

d. Does the grade level fall between 6 and 11 (the one standard deviation range)? <u>No</u>; or between 4 and 13 (the two standard deviation range)? <u>No</u>

3. Looking at grammar

a. For each sentence in the excerpt, underline the <u>subject</u> and double underline the <u>main verb</u>.

b. Fill in Table 1-1, answering the questions for the excerpt's one sentence.

Table 1-1. **Analyze the grammar of the sentence**

Sentence	Does the main verb contain a form of *to be*?	Is the sentence active, passive or neither?	Is the subject abstract or concrete?	Are the subject and verb close together in the first 7–8 words?
1st	yes	active	concrete	no

c. If the subject is abstract, explain, in your own words, why it is abstract.
N/A

4. Prefer the short word

a. Here is a fresh copy of the excerpt. Underline each <u>long word</u>.

In <u>addition</u> to basic research, as part of the <u>Precision</u> <u>Medicine</u> <u>Initiative</u> to <u>encourage</u> more <u>individuals</u> to <u>participate</u> in research studies, the NIH is working with the <u>Department</u> of

Health and Human Services to revise the Common Rule, which is designed to protect research <u>participants</u>, so that more <u>individuals</u> will be <u>eligible</u> to <u>participate</u> in research.

b. Count the number of <u>long words</u> and compute long words as a percent of total words.

<u>12</u> long words/56 total words = <u>21.4</u>%.

c. Double underline any <u>long word</u> you consider a <u>proper name</u> or <u>essential scientific term</u>.

d. For each <u>long word</u> you underlined just once (i.e., skip the essential scientific terms), fill in Table 1-2.

Table 1-2. **Finding shorter words**

Long word	Real world or abstract?	Shorter words that mean about the same thing
addition	abstract	also, too, add, beyond, as well
encourage	abstract	allow, let, inspire, urge, suggest, help, try to get
individuals	real world	people, person, patient, study subject, men and women
participate	abstract?	take part, do, aid, join
participants	real world	people, person, patient, study subject, men and women
eligible	abstract	can, may, allow, get to, qualified, able

e. Look at the long words listed in Table 1-2. Do any of them have the same or a similar meaning?
   - *Encourage and eligible*
   - *Individuals and participants*

f. Fill in Table 1-3 by listing each long word that is a nominalization and giving the root verb or adjective.

Table 1-3. **Find the root verb or adjective for each nominalization**

Nominalization	Root verb or adjective
addition	to add
participants	to participate

5. Looking at meaning and logic

a. Here is another copy of the excerpt. The excerpt answers several basic questions: *Who? What? Why? How? With whom? What for? What else?* Write the question above the part(s) of the sentence that answers that question.

> [*What else?*   ][*How?*   ][
> In addition to basic research, as part of the Precision Medicine Initiative to
>   *Why?*   ][*Who?*][*What?*]
> encourage more individuals to participate in research studies, the NIH is working
> [*With whom?*   ][*What?*   ]
> with the Department of Health and Human Services to revise the Common Rule,
> [*What for?*   ][*Why?*
> which is designed to protect research participants, so that more individuals
>   ]
> will be eligible to participate in research.

b. What is the issue or problem this excerpt deals with?
    Not enough people can take part in research studies, since the Common Rule makes them ineligible.

c. With regard to this issue or problem, does the excerpt: describe it? tell why it is important? offer a solution?
    This excerpt describes the problem, and tells how the NIH is trying to solve it.

d. Does the excerpt frame the issue or problem in real-world terms or abstract terms? Or does it only imply the issue or problem?
    The real-world problem is: a more diverse range of people do not take part in research studies. The abstract problem is: the Common Rule prevents this.

C. Prescription for revising

Write your prescription for revising to treat the symptoms of *medicus incomprehensibilis*. List the things you would recommend to help improve reading ease and clarity.
- *Keep sentence length 15 words average, 25 words maximum*
- *Put the main point first and then give commentary, detail or support*
- *Keep the subject and verb close together in the first 7 or 8 words*
- *Avoid using a high percentage of long words*
- *Keep essential scientific terms; minimize other long words*

D. Revision

Revise the excerpt to improve reading ease and clarity.

> *Beyond doing its basic research, the NIH would like more people to take part in research studies. The NIH is working with the <u>Department</u> of Health and Human Services to revise the Common Rule that protects research subjects. This work is part of the <u>Precision Medicine Initiative</u>.*

1. Looking at WSEG scores

Compute the WSEG score for your revision. Fill in Table 1-4 to show how your revision compares with the original.

Table 1-4. **Comparing WSEG scores**

WSEG		Original	Revised	Change
W	Number of words	56	47	−9
S	Average sentence length	56.0	15.6	−40.4
E	Flesch Reading Ease score	0.0	64.9	64.9
G	Flesch-Kincaid Grade Level	27.3	8.0	−19.3

2. Looking at grammar

Answer the following questions about your revision:

a. Does each sentence put the subject and verb close together within the first 7 or 8 words? If not, tell why it seemed best to do otherwise.
   No. In the first sentence, the subject, "NIH," and verb, "would like," are close together. But the transition phrase, "Beyond doing its basic research," prevents them from being in the first 7 or 8 words.
b. Does each sentence use active voice? If not, tell why it seemed best to do otherwise.
   No. The third sentence is neither active nor passive. It describes a characteristic of the "work," mentioned in the previous sentence.

c. Does each sentence use a concrete subject? If not, tell why it seemed best to use an abstract subject.

No. The third sentence uses an abstract subject, "this work." This nominalization refers back to "working with the Department of Health and Human Services" from the previous sentence.

3. Prefer the short word

a. Underline each <u>long word</u>. Count the number of long words and compute long words as a percent of total words. <u>4</u> long words/<u>47</u> total words = <u>8.5</u>%. Compare your answer with the percent of long words in the original. (See §B.4.b.)

b. Double underline any <u>long word</u> you consider a <u>proper name</u> or <u>essential scientific term</u>.

Note

1. Quoted in Hamilton College, "Writing Tips," https://www.hamilton.edu/tip (accessed October 16, 2016).

2

Finding the Causes of Diarrhoea in Children

Writers in the field of medicine tend to use unfamiliar words in tortuous constructions, particularly when writing reports for submission to learned journals. Research can often be judged only by its final written report. A meticulous study can be let down by poor writing . . . —Neville Goodman and Martin Edwards, *Medical Writing: A Prescription for Clarity*[1]

A. The excerpt

This case study looks at an excerpt from an article published in *The Lancet*.[2] Read the excerpt out loud:

> The increases in estimated burden were a function of improved sensitivity with molecular diagnostics and the higher resolution provided by pathogen quantification. Previous studies of the causes of diarrhoea have generally used non-quantitative diagnostics, which yield dichotomous results at detection limits that might not be clinically relevant. Such results become potentially problematic for the study of causes of diarrhoea in children in resource-limited settings because the rate of enteropathogen carriage shortly after birth is high. *(WSEG = 75/25.0/ 0.0/19.9)*

B. Analyzing the excerpt

1. Initial thoughts

What are some of your initial thoughts on this excerpt?

2. Looking at the WSEG score

a. How does this excerpt's average sentence length compare with the recommended average of 15 words?

b. How many words does each sentence use? First ___, second ___, third ___

c. For each sentence that uses more than 25 words, do you think it needs to be just one long sentence? Why or why not?

d. Does the reading ease score fall between 45 and 70 (the one standard deviation range)?___; or between 33 and 83 (the two standard deviation range)? ____

e. Does the grade level fall between 6 and 11 (the one standard deviation range)? ___; or between 4 and 13 (the two standard deviation range)? ___

3. Looking at grammar

a. For each sentence in the excerpt, underline the subject and double underline the main verb. If the main verb includes a past participle, then draw braces around the {past participle}.

b. Fill in Table 2-1, answering the questions for each sentence.

Table 2-1. **Analyze the grammar of each sentence**

Sentence	Does the main verb contain a form of *to be?*	Is the sentence active, passive or neither?	Is the subject abstract or concrete?	Are the subject and verb close together in the first 7–8 words?
1st				
2nd				
3rd				

c. For each abstract subject, explain, in your own words, why it is abstract.

d. What words or ideas are written in the plural?

e. What words or ideas need to be plural?

f. Fill in Table 2-2 to show your thinking about any phrase that shows possession or connection using *of* or a word ending other than *'s*.

Table 2-2. **Revising phrases to show possession or connection using *of* or a word ending**

List the phrase, underlining of or the word ending	*Is the possession or connection real world or abstract?*	*How might you replace of or the word ending?*

4. Prefer the short word

a. Here is a fresh copy of the excerpt. Underline each long word.

The increases in estimated burden were a function of improved sensitivity with molecular diagnostics and the higher resolution provided by pathogen quantification. Previous studies of the causes of diarrhoea have generally used non-quantitative diagnostics, which yield dichotomous results at detection limits that might not be clinically relevant. Such results become potentially problematic for the study of causes of diarrhoea in children in resource-limited settings because the rate of enteropathogen carriage shortly after birth is high.

b. Count the number of <u>long words</u> and compute long words as a percent of total words.

___ long words/75 total words = ___ %.

c. Double underline any <u>long word</u> you consider a <u>proper name</u> or <u>essential scientific term</u>.

d. For each <u>long word</u> you underlined just once (i.e., skip the essential scientific terms), fill in Table 2-3.

Table 2-3. **Finding shorter words**

Long word	Real world or abstract?	Shorter words that mean about the same thing

e. Look at the long words listed in Table 2-3. Do any of them have the same or a similar meaning?

f. Fill in Table 2-4 by listing each long word that is a nominalization and giving the root verb or adjective.

Table 2-4. **Find the root verb or adjective for each nominalization**

Nominalization	*Root verb or adjective*

g. Does the excerpt use any compound word(s) whose meaning or pronunciation might be clearer if hyphenated or written as an open compound? If so, tell which one(s) and why you think so.

5. Looking at meaning and logic

a. What is the issue or problem this excerpt deals with?

b. With regard to this issue or problem, does the excerpt: describe it? tell why it is important? offer a solution?

c. Does the excerpt frame the issue or problem in real-world terms or abstract terms? Or does it only imply the issue or problem?

C. Prescription for revising

Write your prescription for revising to treat the symptoms of *medicus incomprehensibilis*. List the things you would recommend to help improve reading ease and clarity.

D. Revision

Revise the excerpt to improve reading ease and clarity.

1. Looking at WSEG scores

Compute the WSEG score for your revision. Fill out Table 2-5 to show how your revision compares with the original.

Table 2-5. **Comparing WSEG scores**

WSEG		Original	Revised	Change
W	Number of words	75		
S	Average sentence length	25.0		
E	Flesch Reading Ease score	0.0		
G	Flesch-Kincaid Grade Level	19.9		

2. Looking at grammar

Answer the following questions about your revision:

a. Does each sentence put the subject and verb close together within the first 7 or 8 words? If not, tell why it seemed best to do otherwise.

b. Does each sentence use active voice? If not, tell why it seemed best to do otherwise.

c. Does each sentence use a concrete subject? If not, tell why it seemed best to use an abstract subject.

3. Prefer the short word

a. Underline each <u>long word</u>. Count the number of long words and compute long words as a percent of total words. ＿＿ long words/ ＿＿ total words =＿ %. Compare your answer with the percent of long words in the original. (See §B.4.b.)

b. Double underline any <u>long word</u> you consider a <u>proper name</u> or <u>essential scientific term</u>.

Notes

1. Neville W. Goodman and Martin B. Edwards, *Medical Writing: A Prescription for Clarity*, 4th ed. (Cambridge, UK: Cambridge University Press, 2014), xiii.

2. Jie Liu et al., "Use of Quantitative Molecular Diagnostic Methods to Identify Causes of Diarrhoea in Children: A Reanalysis of the GEMS Case-Control Study," *Lancet* 388, no. 10051 (2016), under "Discussion," http://www.thelancet.com/journals/lancet/article/PIIS0140-6736(16)31529-X/fulltext.

Finding the Causes of Diarrhoea in Children

Never use a long word where a short one will do. —George Orwell,
Politics and the English Language[1]

A. The excerpt

This case study looks at an excerpt from an article published in *The Lancet*. Read the excerpt out loud:

> The <u>increases</u> in estimated burden <u>were</u> a function of improved sensitivity with molecular diagnostics and the higher resolution provided by pathogen quantification. Previous <u>studies</u> of the causes of diarrhoea <u>have</u> generally {<u>used</u>} non-quantitative diagnostics, which yield dichotomous results at detection limits that might not be clinically relevant. Such <u>results</u> <u>become</u> potentially problematic for the study of causes of diarrhoea in children in resource-limited settings because the rate of enteropathogen carriage shortly after birth is high. (*WSEG = 75/25.0/0.0/19.9*)

B. Analyzing the excerpt

1. Initial thoughts

What are some of your initial thoughts on this excerpt?
- *It uses several scientific terms.*
- *It also uses many long words that aren't scientific terms (e.g., generally, potentially, problematic).*

2. Looking at the WSEG score

a. How does this excerpt's average sentence length compare with the recommended average of 15 words?
It has an average sentence length of 25.0 words—more than 1.5 times the recommended average.

b. How many words does each sentence use? First 22, second 25, third 28

c. For each sentence that uses more than 25 words, do you think it needs to be just one long sentence? Why or why not?
The third sentence, which has 28 words, could be broken up into two sentences. We could say, in one sentence, that the results may be a problem. Then, in another sentence, we can tell why.

d. Does the reading ease score fall between 45 and 70 (the one standard deviation range)? *No*; or between 33 and 83 (the two standard deviation range)? *No*

e. Does the grade level fall between 6 and 11 (the one standard deviation range)? *No*; or between 4 and 13 (the two standard deviation range)? *No*

3. Looking at grammar

a. For each sentence in the excerpt, underline the <u>subject</u> and double underline the <u>main verb</u>. If the main verb includes a past participle, then draw braces around the {<u>past participle</u>}.

b. Fill in Table 2-1, answering the questions for each sentence.

Table 2-1. **Analyze the grammar of each sentence**

Sentence	Does the main verb contain a form of to be?	Is the sentence active, passive or neither?	Is the subject abstract or concrete?	Are the subject and verb close together in the first 7–8 words?
1st	yes	neither	abstract	yes
2nd	no	active	abstract	no
3rd	no	active	abstract	yes

c. For each abstract subject, explain, in your own words, why it is abstract.
    - *"Increases (in estimated burden)" describes a conclusion reached through statistical analysis.*
    - *"Studies" involve real-world activities guided by abstract thought and analysis.*
    - *"Results" involve conclusions drawn from analysis.*
d. What words or ideas are written in the plural?
    Increases, diagnostics, studies, causes, results, limits, children, settings
e. What words or ideas need to be plural?
    Diagnostics, studies, results, limits, children, settings
f. Fill in Table 2-2 to show your thinking about any phrase that shows possession or connection using *of* or a word ending other than *'s*.

Table 2-2. **Revising phrases to show possession or connection using *of* or a word ending**

List the phrase, underlining <u>of</u> or the <u>word ending</u>	Is the possession or connection real world or abstract?	How might you replace of or the word ending?
function <u>of</u> improved sensitivity with molecul<u>ar</u> diagnostics	*abstract*	*due to molecul<u>ar</u> diagnostics*
previous studies <u>of</u> the causes <u>of</u> diarrhoea	*studies—abstract; causes of diarrhoea—real world*	*previous studies on what causes diarrhoea*
dichotom<u>ous</u> results	*abstract*	*differing results*
rate <u>of</u> enteropathogen carriage	*abstract*	*(no change)*

4. Prefer the short word

a. Here is a fresh copy of the excerpt. Underline each long word.

> The increases in <u>estimated</u> burden were a function of improved <u>sensitivity</u> with <u>molecular</u> <u>diagnostics</u> and the higher <u>resolution</u> provided by <u>pathogen</u> <u>quantification</u>. <u>Previous</u> studies of the causes of <u>diarrhoea</u> have <u>generally</u> used <u>non-quantitative</u> <u>diagnostics</u>, which yield <u>dichotomous</u> results at <u>detection</u> limits that might not be <u>clinically</u> <u>relevant</u>. Such results become <u>potentially</u> <u>problematic</u> for the study of causes of <u>diarrhoea</u> in children in <u>resource-limited</u> settings because the rate of <u>enteropathogen</u> carriage shortly after birth is high.

b. Count the number of <u>long words</u> and compute long words as a percent of total words.

<u>21</u> long words/75 total words = <u>28.0</u>%.

c. Double underline any <u>long word</u> you consider a <u>proper name</u> or <u>essential scientific term</u>.

d. For each <u>long word</u> you underlined just once (i.e., skip the essential scientific terms), fill in Table 2-3.

Table 2-3. **Finding shorter words**

Long word	Real world or abstract?	Shorter words that mean about the same thing
estimated	abstract	predicted, likely, expect, guess
sensitivity	abstract	sensitive, correct, better data
resolution	abstract	resolve, clear, clarity, optics, vision, see, focus
pathogen	real world	germ, bug, virus
quantification	abstract	count, number, quantify, quantity
previous	abstract	past, other, before, early, former, last
generally	abstract	often, most often, most of the time, almost all, almost always, many, as a rule, in general
non-quantitative	abstract	not quantitative, not able to quantify, cannot count, not counted, uncountable, unknown number, unknown quantity
dichotomous	abstract	divided, in two parts, two-part, differing, split
detection	abstract	detect, find, able to see
clinically	abstract	clinical, in practice, treat a patient, examine a patient
relevant	abstract	fitting, proper, useful, relate, fit, suits
potentially	abstract	likely, possibly, probably, may, could be, possible
problematic	abstract	problem, issue, tricky, difficult, hard, not helpful
resource-limited (setting)	abstract	limited resources, scarce resources, poverty, scarcity, poor, destitute, not rich
enteropathogen	real world	gut pathogen, germs in the gut, gut bacteria, bacteria

e. Look at the long words listed in Table 2-3. Do any of them have the same or a similar meaning?
    - *Sensitivity and detection*
    - *Pathogen and enteropathogen*
f. Fill in Table 2-4 by listing each long word that is a nominalization and giving the root verb or adjective.

Table 2-4. **Find the root verb or adjective for each nominalization**

Nominalization	Root verb or adjective
sensitivity	to sense, sensitive
resolution	to resolve
quantification	to quantify
detection	to detect

g. Does the excerpt use any compound word(s) whose meaning or pronunciation might be clearer if hyphenated or written as an open compound? If so, tell which one(s) and why you think so.
    We would prefer to hyphenate "entero-pathogen," so a reader can better see the two parts.

5. Looking at meaning and logic

a. What is the issue or problem this excerpt deals with?
    What caused the increase in estimated burden of diarrhoea in children?
b. With regard to this issue or problem, does the excerpt: describe it? tell why it is important? offer a solution?
    It offers a solution (i.e., an explanation): the increase in the estimated burden is due to using molecular diagnostics, a new, more sensitive process.
c. Does the excerpt frame the issue or problem in real-world terms or abstract terms? Or does it only imply the issue or problem?
    The issue is framed in abstract terms—as "increases in estimated burden." The excerpt seems to say, the increase in estimated burden does not necessarily correspond to an increase in diarrhoea in children.

C. Prescription for revising

Write your prescription for revising to treat the symptoms of *medicus incomprehensibilis*. List the things you would recommend to help improve reading ease and clarity.
- *Keep sentence length 15 words average, 25 words maximum*
- *Revise abstract into concrete*
- *Keep the subject and verb close together in the first 7 or 8 words*
- *Omit the needless of*
- *Keep essential scientific terms; minimize other long words*
- *Prefer the short word to talk about the real world*
- *Convert nominalization into a verb in active voice*

D. Revision

Revise the excerpt to improve reading ease and clarity.

> *The rise in the predicted burden of <u>diarrhoea</u> is due to a more <u>sensitive</u> process: <u>molecular diagnostics</u>. This process allows us to better see and count the <u>pathogens</u>. Most past studies could not do this. This gave differing results at <u>detection</u> limits, which might not be helpful when treating a patient. These results might cause a problem when studying children in poor areas since, just after birth, the number of gut <u>pathogens</u> is high.*

1. Looking at WSEG scores

Compute the WSEG score for your revision. Fill out Table 2-5 to show how your revision compares with the original.

Table 2-5. **Comparing WSEG scores**

WSEG		*Original*	*Revised*	*Change*
W	Number of words	75	74	−1
S	Average sentence length	25.0	14.8	−10.2
E	Flesch Reading Ease score	0.0	62.6	62.6
G	Flesch-Kincaid Grade Level	19.9	8.2	−11.7

2. Looking at grammar

Answer the following questions about your revision:

a. Does each sentence put the subject and verb close together within the first 7 or 8 words? If not, tell why it seemed best to do otherwise.
   No. In the first sentence, the subject, "rise," and verb, "is due," are separated by the long logical subject, "The rise in the predicted burden of diarrhoea."

b. Does each sentence use active voice? If not, tell why it seemed best to do otherwise.
   No. The first sentence is neither active nor passive. This tracks the original.

c. Does each sentence use a concrete subject? If not, tell why it seemed best to use an abstract subject.
   No. We used a number of abstract subjects:

   - *The first sentence of the original used an abstract subject, "the increases in estimated burden," which apparently refers back to the previous paragraph. Therefore, we felt we should keep the same abstract subject in our first sentence. However, we did change the word "increases" to "rise."*
   - *In the second, third, and fourth sentences, we used the abstract subjects "this" and "these" to continue the idea from the previous sentence.*

3. Prefer the short word

a. Underline each <u>long word</u>. Count the number of long words and compute long words as a percent of total words. <u>7</u> long words/<u>74</u> total words = <u>9.5</u>%. Compare your answer with the percent of long words in the original. (See §B.4.b.)

b. Double underline any <u>long word</u> you consider a <u>proper name</u> or <u>essential scientific term</u>.

Note

1. George Orwell, "Politics and the English Language," *Horizon* 13, no. 76 (1964), https://biblio.wiki/index.php?title=Politics_and_the_English_Language&oldid=63964 (accessed January 19, 2018).

3

Trends in Adult Body-Mass Index

Jargon has its place, . . . but jargon can become a 'secret' language
excluding people outside of the expert group. When you aim to
communicate beyond the expert group, plain language can help reach
an audience that is very broad in terms of experience, education,
and interest. —Primary Health Care Research & Information
Service (Australia)[1]

A. The excerpt

This case study looks at an excerpt from an article published in *The Lancet.*[2]
Read the excerpt out loud:

> High body-mass index (BMI) is an important risk factor for cardio-
> vascular and kidney diseases, diabetes, some cancers, and musculo-
> skeletal disorders. Concerns about the health and economic burden of
> increasing BMI have led to adiposity being included among the global
> non-communicable disease (NCD) targets, with a target of halting, by
> 2025, the rise in the prevalence of obesity at its 2010 level. Information
> on whether countries are on track to achieve this target is needed to
> support accountability towards the global NCD commitments. (*WSEG*
> *= 82/27.3/12.9/18.2)*

B. Analyzing the excerpt

1. Initial thoughts

What are some of your initial thoughts on this excerpt?

2. Looking at the WSEG score

a. How does this excerpt's average sentence length compare with the recommended average of 15 words?

b. How many words does each sentence use? First ____, second____, third ____

c. For each sentence that uses more than 25 words, do you think it needs to be just one long sentence? Why or why not?

d. Does the reading ease score fall between 45 and 70 (the one standard deviation range)?____; or between 33 and 83 (the two standard deviation range)? ____

e. Does the grade level fall between 6 and 11 (the one standard deviation range)?____; or between 4 and 13 (the two standard deviation range)? ____

3. Looking at grammar

a. For each sentence in the excerpt, underline the subject and double underline the main verb. If the main verb includes a past participle, then draw braces around the {past participle}.

b. Fill in Table 3-1, answering the questions for each sentence.

Table 3-1. **Analyze the grammar of each sentence**

Sentence	Does the main verb contain a form of to be?	Is the sentence active, passive or neither?	Is the subject abstract or concrete?	Are the subject and verb close together in the first 7–8 words?
1st				
2nd				
3rd				

c. For each abstract subject, explain, in your own words, why it is abstract.

d. What words or ideas are written in the plural?

e. What words or ideas need to be plural?

f. Fill in Table 3-2 to show your thinking about any phrase that shows possession or connection using *of* or a word ending other than *'s*.

Table 3-2. **Revising phrases that show possession or connection using *of* or a word ending**

List the phrase, underlining of or the word ending	*Is the possession or connection real world or abstract?*	*How might you replace of or the word ending?*

4. Prefer the short word

a. Here is a fresh copy of the excerpt. Underline each <u>long word</u>.

> High body-mass index (BMI) is an important risk factor for cardiovascular and kidney diseases, diabetes, some cancers, and musculoskeletal disorders. Concerns about the health and economic burden of increasing BMI have led to adiposity being included among the global non-communicable disease (NCD) targets, with a target of halting, by 2025, the rise in the prevalence of obesity at its 2010 level. Information on whether countries are on track to achieve this target is needed to support accountability towards the global NCD commitments.

b. Count the number of <u>long words</u> and compute long words as a percent of total words.
_____ long words/82 total words = _____ %.

c. Double underline any <u>long word</u> you consider a <u>proper name</u> or <u>essential scientific term</u>.

d. For each <u>long word</u> you underlined just once (i.e., skip the essential scientific terms), fill in Table 3-3.

Table 3-3. **Finding shorter words**

Long word	Real world or abstract?	Shorter words that mean about the same thing

e. Look at the long words listed in Table 3-3. Do any of them have the same or a similar meaning?

f. Fill in Table 3-4 by listing each long word that is a nominalization and giving the root verb or adjective.

Table 3-4. **Find the root verb or adjective for each nominalization**

Nominalization	Root verb or adjective

g. Does the excerpt use any compound word(s) whose meaning or pronunciation might be clearer if hyphenated or written as an open compound? If so, tell which one(s) and why you think so.

5. Looking at meaning and logic

a. What is the issue or problem this excerpt deals with?

b. With regard to this issue or problem, does the excerpt: describe it? tell why it is important? offer a solution?

c. Does the excerpt frame the issue or problem in real-world terms or abstract terms? Or does it only imply the issue or problem?

d. What types of people might want to read an article about the rise in obesity worldwide? In other words, who is the widest reasonable audience? Would you recommend any changes to help make this excerpt clearer for the widest reasonable audience?

C. Prescription for revising

Write your prescription for revising to treat the symptoms of *medicus incomprehensibilis*. List the things you would recommend to help improve reading ease and clarity.

D. Revision

Revise the excerpt to improve reading ease and clarity.

1. Looking at WSEG scores

Compute the WSEG score for your revision. Fill in Table 3-5 to show how your revision compares with the original.

Table 3-5. **Comparing WSEG scores**

WSEG		Original	Revised	Change
W	Number of words	82		
S	Average sentence length	27.3		
E	Flesch Reading Ease score	12.9		
G	Flesch-Kincaid Grade Level	18.2		

2. Looking at grammar

Answer the following questions about your revision:

a. Does each sentence put the subject and verb close together within the first 7 or 8 words? If not, tell why it seemed best to do otherwise.

b. Does each sentence use active voice? If not, tell why it seemed best to do otherwise.

c. Does each sentence use a concrete subject? If not, tell why it seemed best to use an abstract subject.

3. Prefer the short word

a. Underline each <u>long word</u>. Count the number of long words and compute long words as a percent of total words. ___ long words /___ total words = ___ %. Compare your answer with the percent of long words in the original. (See §B.4.b.)

b. Double underline any <u>long word</u> you consider a <u>proper name</u> or <u>essential scientific term</u>.

Notes

1. Primary Health Care Research & Information Service, "Introduction to Plain Language," http://www.phcris.org.au/guides/plain_language.php (accessed January 3, 2018).
2. NCD Risk Factor Collaboration, "Trends in Adult Body-Mass Index in 200 Countries from 1975 to 2014: A Pooled Analysis of 1698 Population-Based Measurement Studies in 19.2 Million Participants," *Lancet* 387, no. 10026 (April 2016), under "Introduction," http://www.thelancet.com/journals/lancet/article/PIIS0140-6736(16)30054-X/fulltext.

Trends in Adult Body-Mass Index

Vagueness can result from uncertainty, from the mental haze of abstract thought, or a worm in the brain that makes one yearn for official-sounding prose. . . . If you can give a down-to-earth description, you'll be writing better. Try to convey a mental image of what you describe. —Bryan A. Garner[1]

A. The excerpt

This case study looks at an excerpt from an article published in *The Lancet*. Read the excerpt out loud:

> High <u>body-mass index</u> (BMI) <u>is</u> an important risk factor for cardio-vascular and kidney diseases, diabetes, some cancers, and musculo-skeletal disorders. <u>Concerns</u> about the health and economic burden of increasing BMI <u>have {led}</u> to adiposity being included among the global non-communicable disease (NCD) targets, with a target of halting, by 2025, the rise in the prevalence of obesity at its 2010 level. <u>Information</u> on whether countries are on track to achieve this target <u>is {needed}</u> to support accountability towards the global NCD commitments. (*WSEG = 82/27.3/12.9/18.2*)

B. Analyzing the excerpt

1. Initial thoughts

What are some of your initial thoughts on this excerpt?

- *The excerpt uses several related terms: high body-mass index, BMI, increasing BMI, adiposity, obesity. Is this elegant variation?*
- *The first sentence covers two ideas: What is BMI? and, If a person has a high BMI, for what diseases are they at risk?*
- *It is also awkward since BMI stands for "body mass index," not "<u>high</u> body mass index."*
- *The real-world risk factor is excess body fat. BMI is a math calculation used to measure body fat.*
- *The second sentence seems very long and contains two distinct ideas.*

2. Looking at the WSEG score

a. How does this excerpt's average sentence length compare with the recommended average of 15 words?
    The average sentence length is 27.3 words—nearly twice the recommended average.

b. How many words does each sentence use? First <u>20</u>, second <u>41</u>, third <u>21</u>

c. For each sentence that uses more than 25 words, do you think it needs to be just one long sentence? Why or why not?
    The second sentence, which uses 41 words, could be broken up into two sentences. We could say, in one sentence, that obesity has been added to the list of NCD targets. Then, in another sentence, we could explain the target for obesity.

d. Does the reading ease score fall between 45 and 70 (the one standard deviation range)? <u>*No*</u>; or between 33 and 83 (the two standard deviation range)? <u>*No*</u>

e. Does the grade level fall between 6 and 11 (the one standard deviation range)? <u>*No*</u>; or between 4 and 13 (the two standard deviation range)? <u>*No*</u>

3. Looking at grammar

a. For each sentence in the excerpt, underline the <u>subject</u> and double underline the <u>main verb</u>. If the main verb includes a past participle, then draw braces around the {<u>past participle</u>}.

b. Fill in Table 3-1, answering the questions for each sentence.

Table 3-1. **Analyze the grammar of each sentence**

Sentence	Does the main verb contain a form of *to be*?	Is the sentence active, passive or neither?	Is the subject abstract or concrete?	Are the subject and verb close together in the first 7–8 words?
1st	yes	neither	abstract	yes
2nd	no	active	abstract	no
3rd	yes	passive	abstract	no

c. For each abstract subject, explain, in your own words, why it is abstract.
   - *"Body-mass index" involves a math calculation based on height and weight.*
   - *"Concerns" involve thoughts or emotions.*
   - *"Information" refers to facts, ideas or knowledge.*

d. What words or ideas are written in the plural?

Diseases, cancers, disorders, concerns, targets, countries, commitments

e. What words or ideas need to be plural?

Diseases, cancers, disorders, concerns, targets

f. Fill in Table 3-2 to show your thinking about any phrase that shows possession or connection using *of* or a word ending other than *'s*.

Table 3-2. **Revising phrases that show possession or connection using *of* or a word ending**

List the phrase, underlining *of* or the <u>word ending</u>	Is the possession or connection real world or abstract?	How might you replace *of* or the word ending?
cardiovascular and kidney diseases	*real world*	*heart, blood vessel and kidney diseases*
musculoskeletal disorders	*real world*	*muscle and skeletal disorders*
concerns about the health and economic burden of increasing BMI	*abstract*	*concerns about rising obesity*
target of halting	*abstract*	*a goal to stop*
prevalence of obesity	*abstract*	*obesity*

4. Prefer the short word

a. Here is a fresh copy of the excerpt. Underline each <u>long word</u>.

> High <u>body-mass</u> index (BMI) is an <u>important</u> risk factor for <u>cardiovascular</u> and kidney diseases, <u>diabetes</u>, some cancers, and <u>musculoskeletal</u> <u>disorders</u>. Concerns about the health and <u>economic</u> burden of increasing BMI have led to <u>adiposity</u> being included among the global <u>non-communicable</u> disease (NCD) targets, with a target of halting, by 2025, the rise in the <u>prevalence</u> of <u>obesity</u> at its 2010 level. <u>Information</u> on whether countries are on track to achieve this target is needed to support <u>accountability</u> towards the global NCD <u>commitments</u>.

b. Count the number of <u>long words</u> and compute long words as a percent of total words.

<u>14</u> long words/82 total words = <u>17.1</u>%.

c. Double underline any <u>long word</u> you consider a <u>proper name</u> or <u>essential scientific term</u>.

d. For each <u>long word</u> you underlined just once (i.e., skip the essential scientific terms), fill in Table 3-3.

Table 3-3. **Finding shorter words**

Long word	Real world or abstract?	Shorter words that mean about the same thing
body-mass	real world	body mass
important	abstract	big, major, great, large, crucial, key
cardiovascular	real world	heart and blood vessels
musculoskeletal	real world	muscle and skeleton
disorders	real world	disease, illness
economic	abstract	economy, money, finance
adiposity	real world	obese, obesity, excess body fat, fatness
non-communicable	real world	non-infectious, not infectious, cannot share, cannot catch
prevalence	abstract	number of, people with
obesity	real world	excess body fat, fatness, obese, BMI ≥30
information	abstract	facts, data, report
accountability	abstract	to be accountable, to track, on track, progress
commitments	abstract	goals, pledge, duty, promise, vow

e. Look at the long words listed in Table 3-3. Do any of them have the same or a similar meaning?

Body-mass, adiposity and obesity

f. Fill in Table 3-4 by listing each long word that is a nominalization and giving the root verb or adjective.

Table 3-4. **Find the root verb or adjective for each nominalization**

Nominalization	Root verb or adjective
disorders	to (dis-) order
prevalence	to prevail
information	to inform
accountability	to account, able
commitments	to commit

g. Does the excerpt use any compound word(s) whose meaning or pronunciation might be clearer if hyphenated or written as an open compound? If so, tell which one(s) and why you think so.
We would write "body mass" as an open compound. It is commonly written this way and the word is clear without hyphenation. We might hyphenate "cardiovascular" and "musculo-skeletal," so the reader can better see the two parts.

5. Looking at meaning and logic

a. What is the issue or problem this excerpt deals with?
Obesity is rising worldwide. Data is needed on whether each country is on track to reach their target for controlling obesity.

b. With regard to this issue or problem, does the excerpt: describe it? tell why it is important? offer a solution?
The excerpt tells what the problem is (rising BMI), why it is important (because it is an important risk factor), and some steps for solving it (adding adiposity to the list of NCD targets).

c. Does the excerpt frame the issue or problem in real-world terms or abstract terms? Or does it only imply the issue or problem?
The excerpt talks about the problem in abstract terms (i.e., BMI, adiposity, obesity, risk factor) and avoids real-world terms (i.e., excess body fat).

d. What types of people might want to read an article about the rise in obesity worldwide? In other words, who is the widest reasonable audience? Would you recommend any changes to help make this excerpt clearer for the widest reasonable audience?

The widest reasonable audience for this article includes journal subscribers, doctors who treat patients who have a high BMI, nurses, nutritionists, weight loss practitioners, chiropractors, public health officials, statisticians, economists, and politicians. This would include people at all levels of training and around the world.

Considering this wide audience, we think not everyone would know what BMI is, how it is measured, and how obesity and BMI are related. Therefore, we would add a few sentences to explain these concepts.

C. Prescription for revising

Write your prescription for revising to treat the symptoms of *medicus incomprehensibilis*. List the things you would recommend to help improve reading ease and clarity.

- *Keep sentence length 15 words average, 25 words maximum*
- *Minimize forms of to be*
- *Revise passive into active voice*
- *Revise abstract into concrete*
- *Observe the 1066 principle*
- *Keep the subject and verb close together in the first 7 or 8 words*
- *Keep essential scientific terms; minimize other long words*
- *Prefer the short word to describe the real world*
- *Use terms consistently; avoid elegant variation*
- *Convert nominalization into a verb in active voice*
- *Start by anchoring the discussion in the real world*
- *Explain each step of reasoning*

D. Revision

Revise the excerpt to improve reading ease and clarity.

Excess body fat puts a person at risk for many diseases. This includes <u>diabetes</u>, some cancers, and heart and blood vessel, kidney, and muscle and <u>skeletal</u> diseases. Body fat is <u>estimated</u> using the body mass index (BMI), which equals weight (kg) divided by height squared (m^2). A person is deemed "obese" if they have a BMI of 30 or more.

<u>Obesity</u> is rising worldwide. Concerns about this trend have led to <u>obesity</u> being included among the global <u>non-infectious</u> disease (NID) targets. The goal is to halt the rise in <u>obesity</u>, keep it at its 2010 level, and do this by 2025. Data is needed on whether each country is on track to achieve this goal.

1. Looking at WSEG scores

Compute the WSEG score for your revision. Fill in Table 3-5 to show how your revision compares with the original.

Table 3-5. **Comparing WSEG scores**

WSEG		Original	Revised	Change
W	Number of words	82	115	33
S	Average sentence length	27.3	14.3	–13.0
E	Flesch Reading Ease score	12.9	59.8	46.9
G	Flesch-Kincaid Grade Level	18.2	8.4	–9.8

2. Looking at grammar

Answer the following questions about your revision:

a. Does each sentence put the subject and verb close together within the first 7 or 8 words? If not, tell why it seemed best to do otherwise.
Yes.

b. Does each sentence use active voice? If not, tell why it seemed best to do otherwise.
No. A few sentences use passive voice.
   - *Paragraph 1, the third and fourth sentences are passive. Estimating a patient's level of body fat is important; but who does the estimation is not. Similarly, knowing what BMI level constitutes "obesity" is important; but who made this decision is not.*
   - *Paragraph 2, the third sentence is neither active nor passive. The fact that obesity has been included in the NID targets is important; but exactly who decided this is not.*
   - *Paragraph 2, the last sentence is passive. Data about whether countries are on track to meet their targets is needed; who might provide this data remains unclear.*

c. Does each sentence use a concrete subject? If not, tell why it seemed best to use an abstract subject.
No. The original excerpt discussed the abstract subject of BMI and related concerns and data. In our revision, we started by talking about excess body fat, the real-world medical problem. Once we did this, we followed the original thread of discussion by talking about the problem in abstract terms.

3. Prefer the short word

a. Underline each <u>long word</u>. Count the number of long words and compute long words as a percent of total words. <u>7</u> long words/<u>115</u> total words = <u>6.1</u>%. Compare your answer with the percent of long words in the original. (See §B.4.b.)

b. Double underline any <u>long word</u> you consider a <u>proper name</u> or <u>essential scientific term</u>.

4. Additional comments

Why did our revision use 33 more words than the original?

We thought the original left out two steps of logic that the widest reasonable audience might need to understand the excerpt. We added sentences to tell what BMI is and how it is calculated.

Note

1. Bryan A. Garner, *The Redbook: A Manual of Legal Style* (St. Paul, MN: Thomson West, 2006), sec. 13.4. The parenthetical statements and legal examples have been omitted.

Herniated Lumbar Inter-Vertebral Disk

The Times of India has won one of the world's leading media awards for simple and effective use of the English language. . . . In November, [The Times of India] front-paged a report asking if it were time to do away with Latin jargon such as suo moto, vis-à-vis, quid pro quo, and inter alia to allow more English-speaking Indians to understand what's being said. The report argued that because English is not our first language, we should make it simpler and more people-friendly. —Times of India[1]

A. The excerpt

This case study looks at an excerpt from an article published in *The New England Journal of Medicine*.[2] Read the excerpt out loud:

> In patients with acute disk herniations, avoidance of prolonged inactivity in order to prevent debilitation is important. Most patients can be encouraged to stand and walk. The ability to sit comfortably is a sign of improvement in the patient's condition and suggests that more structured exercise can be undertaken. Evidence regarding the effects of physical therapy and exercise is limited. A systematic review of five randomized trials showed that patients who participated in supervised exercise had greater short-term pain relief than patients who received counseling alone, but this reduction in pain was small and these patients did not have a long-term benefit with respect to reduced pain or disability. *(WSEG = 109/21.8/29.4/14.5)*

B. Analyzing the excerpt

1. Initial thoughts

What are some of your initial thoughts on this excerpt?

2. Looking at the WSEG score

a. How does this excerpt's average sentence length compare with the recommended average of 15 words?

b. Count the number of words in each sentence. Then calculate the total number of words. Write your answers in Table 4-1.

Table 4-1. **Words per sentence**

	Sentence					
	1st	2nd	3rd	4th	5th	Total
Number of words						

c. For each sentence that uses more than 25 words, do you think it needs to be just one long sentence? Why or why not?

d. Does the reading ease score fall between 45 and 70 (the one standard deviation range)? ___; or between 33 and 83 (the two standard deviation range)? ___

e. Does the grade level fall between 6 and 11 (the one standard deviation range)?___; or between 4 and 13 (the two standard deviation range)? ___

3. Looking at grammar

a. For each sentence in the excerpt, underline the <u>subject</u> and double underline the <u>main verb</u>. If the main verb includes a past participle, then draw braces around the {<u>past participle</u>}.

b. Fill in Table 4-2, answering the questions for each sentence.

Table 4-2. **Analyze the grammar of each sentence**

Sentence	*Does the main verb contain a form of* to be?	*Is the sentence active, passive or neither?*	*Is the subject abstract or concrete?*	*Are the subject and verb close together in the first 7–8 words?*
1st				
2nd				
3rd				
4th				
5th				

c. For each abstract subject, explain, in your own words, why it is abstract.

d. What words or ideas are written in the plural?

e. What words or ideas need to be plural?

f. Fill in Table 4-3 to show your thinking about any phrase that shows possession or connection using *of* or a word ending other than *'s*.

Table 4-3. **Revising phrases that show possession or connection using *of* or a word ending**

List the phrase, underlining of *or the* word ending	*Is the possession or connection real world or abstract?*	*How might you replace* of *or the word ending?*

4. Prefer the short word

a. Here is a fresh copy of the excerpt. Underline each <u>long word</u>.

> In patients with acute disk herniations, avoidance of prolonged inactivity in order to prevent debilitation is important. Most patients can be encouraged to stand and walk. The ability to sit comfortably is a sign of improvement in the patient's condition and suggests that more structured exercise can be undertaken. Evidence regarding the effects of physical therapy and exercise is limited. A systematic review of five randomized trials showed that patients who participated in supervised exercise had greater short-term pain relief than patients who received counseling alone, but this reduction in pain was small and these patients did not have a long-term benefit with respect to reduced pain or disability.

b. Count the number of <u>long words</u> and compute long words as a percent of total words.
    ___ long words/109 total words = ___ %.

c. Double underline any <u>long word</u> you consider a <u>proper name</u> or <u>essential scientific term</u>.

d. For each <u>long word</u> you underlined just once (i.e., skip the essential scientific terms), fill in Table 4-4.

Table 4-4. **Finding shorter words**

Long word	Real world or abstract?	Shorter words that mean about the same thing

Long word	Real world or abstract?	Shorter words that mean about the same thing

e. Look at the long words listed in Table 4-4. Do any of them have the same or a similar meaning?

f. Fill in Table 4-5 by listing each long word that is a nominalization and giving the root verb or adjective.

Table 4-5. **Find the root verb or adjective for each nominalization**

Nominalization	Root verb or adjective

g. Does the excerpt use any compound word(s) whose meaning or pronunciation might be clearer if hyphenated or written as an open compound? If so, tell which one(s) and why you think so.

5. Looking at meaning and logic

a. What is the issue or problem this excerpt deals with?

b. With regard to this issue or problem, does the excerpt: describe it? tell why it's important? offer a solution?

c. Does the excerpt frame the issue or problem in real-world terms or abstract terms? Or does it only imply the issue or problem?

C. Prescription for revising

Write your prescription for revising to treat the symptoms of *medicus incomprehensibilis*. List the things you would recommend to help improve reading ease and clarity.

D. Revision

Revise the excerpt to improve reading ease and clarity.

1. Looking at *WSEG* scores

Compute the *WSEG* score for your revision. Fill in Table 4-6 to show how your revision compares with the original.

Table 4-6. **Comparing *WSEG* scores**

WSEG		*Original*	*Revised*	*Change*
W	Number of words	109		
S	Average sentence length	21.8		
E	Flesch Reading Ease score	29.4		
G	Flesch-Kincaid Grade Level	14.5		

2. Looking at grammar

Answer the following questions about your revision:

a. Does each sentence put the subject and verb close together within the first 7 or 8 words? If not, tell why it seemed best to do otherwise.

b. Does each sentence use active voice? If not, tell why it seemed best to do otherwise.

   c. Does each sentence use a concrete subject? If not, tell why it seemed best to use an abstract subject.

3. Prefer the short word

   a. Underline each <u>long word</u>. Count the number of <u>long words</u> and compute long words as a percent of total words. ___ long words / ___ total words = ___ %. Compare your answer with the percent of long words in the original. (See §B.4.b.)

   b. Double underline any <u>long word</u> you consider a <u>proper name</u> or <u>essential scientific term</u>.

Notes

1. Times News Network (TNN), "TOI Wins Global Award for Plain English," *Times of India,* February 13, 2009. http://timesofindia.indiatimes.com/india/TOI-wins-global-award-for-plain-English/articleshow/4124976.cms (accessed January 3, 2018).
2. Richard A. Deyo and Sphail K. Mirza, "Herniated Lumbar Intervertebral Disk." *N Engl J Med* 374, no. 18 (2016): 1768.

Herniated Lumbar Inter-Vertebral Disk

When you are talking to your reader, say exactly what you mean, using the simplest words that fit. This does not necessarily mean only using simple words— just words that the reader will understand. —Plain English Campaign (UK), *How to Write in Plain English*[1]

A. The excerpt

This case study looks at an excerpt from an article published in *The New England Journal of Medicine.* Read the excerpt out loud:

> In patients with acute disk herniations, <u>avoidance</u> of prolonged inactivity in order to prevent debilitation <u>is</u> important. Most <u>patients</u> <u>can</u> <u>be</u> {<u>encouraged</u>} to stand and walk. The <u>ability</u> to sit comfortably <u>is</u> a sign of improvement in the patient's condition and suggests that more structured exercise can be undertaken. <u>Evidence</u> regarding the effects of physical therapy and exercise <u>is</u> {<u>limited</u>}. A systematic <u>review</u> of five randomized trials <u>showed</u> that patients who participated in supervised exercise had greater short-term pain relief than patients who received counseling alone, but this reduction in pain was small and these patients did not have a long-term benefit with respect to reduced pain or disability. *(WSEG = 109/21.8/29.4/14.5)*

B. Analyzing the excerpt

1. Initial thoughts

What are some of your initial thoughts on this excerpt?
- *The excerpt talks about patients in the plural (rather than one typical patient).*
- *It uses several nominalizations (e.g., herniations, avoidance, inactivity).*
- *A few sentences use passive voice.*
- *The last sentence is very long.*

2. Looking at the WSEG score

a. How does this excerpt's average sentence length compare with the recommended average of 15 words?
   The average sentence length is 21.8 words—a little less than 1.5 times the recommended average.

b. Count the number of words in each sentence. Then calculate the total number of words. Write your answers in Table 4-1.

Table 4-1. **Words per sentence**

	Sentence					
	1st	*2nd*	*3rd*	*4th*	*5th*	*Total*
Number of words	17	9	23	11	49	109

c. For each sentence that uses more than 25 words, do you think it needs to be just one long sentence? Why or why not?
   The last sentence, which has 49 words, could be broken up into a few sentences. We could say, in one sentence, what the review of randomized trials showed. In another sentence, we could say how exercise helps to reduce short-term pain. Then, in yet another sentence, we could tell about the long-term effects.

d. Does the reading ease score fall between 45 and 70 (the one standard deviation range)? <u>No</u>; or between 33 and 83 (the two standard deviation range)? <u>No</u>

e. Does the grade level fall between 6 and 11 (the one standard deviation range)? <u>No</u>; or between 4 and 13 (the two standard deviation range)? <u>No</u>

3. Looking at grammar

a. For each sentence in the excerpt, underline the <u>subject</u> and double underline the <u>main verb</u>. If the main verb includes a past participle, then draw braces around the {<u>past participle</u>}.

b. Fill in Table 4-2, answering the questions for each sentence.

Table 4-2. **Analyze the grammar of each sentence**

Sentence	*Does the main verb contain a form of to be?*	*Is the sentence active, passive or neither?*	*Is the subject abstract or concrete?*	*Are the subject and verb close together in the first 7–8 words?*
1st	yes	neither	abstract	no
2nd	yes	passive	concrete	yes
3rd	yes	neither	abstract	yes
4th	yes	neither	abstract	no
5th	no	active	abstract	yes

c. For each abstract subject, explain, in your own words, why it is abstract.
  - *"Avoidance" means intentionally not doing something.*
  - *"Ability" indicates the potential to act in the real world, but not necessarily real-world action.*
  - *"Evidence" relates to analyzing research articles or patient charts.*
  - *"Review" involves analyzing information.*

d. What words or ideas are written in the plural?
  Patients, herniations, effects, trials

e. What words or ideas need to be plural?
  Trials

f. Fill in Table 4-3 to show your thinking about any phrase that shows possession or connection using *of* or a word ending other than *'s*.

Table 4-3. **Revising phrases that show possession or connection using *of* or a word ending**

List the phrase, underlining of or the word ending	*Is the possession or connection real world or abstract?*	*How might you replace of or the word ending?*
avoid<u>ance</u> <u>of</u> prolonged inactivity	abstract	*avoid prolonged inactivity*
sign <u>of</u> improvement	real world	*sign they are improving*
effects <u>of</u> physical therapy and exercise	real world	*(no change)*
systemat<u>ic</u> review <u>of</u> five randomized trials	abstract	*(no change)*

4. Prefer the short word

a. Here is a fresh copy of the excerpt. Underline each long word.

> In patients with acute disk <u>herniations,</u> <u>avoidance</u> of prolonged <u>inactivity</u> in order to prevent <u>debilitation</u> is <u>important.</u> Most patients can be <u>encouraged</u> to stand and walk. The <u>ability</u> to sit <u>comfortably</u> is a sign of <u>improvement</u> in the patient's <u>condition</u> and suggests that more structured <u>exercise</u> can be <u>undertaken.</u> <u>Evidence</u> regarding the effects of <u>physical</u> <u>therapy</u> and <u>exercise</u> is limited. A <u>systematic</u> review of five <u>randomized</u> trials showed that patients who <u>participated</u> in <u>supervised</u> <u>exercise</u> had greater short-term pain relief than patients who received counseling alone, but this <u>reduction</u> in pain was small and these patients did not have a long-term <u>benefit</u> with respect to reduced pain or <u>disability.</u>

b. Count the number of <u>long words</u> and compute long words as a percent of total words.
   <u>24</u> long words/109 total words = <u>22.0%</u>

c. Double underline any <u>long word</u> you consider a <u>proper name</u> or <u>essential scientific term</u>.

d. For each <u>long word</u> you underlined just once (i.e., skip the essential scientific terms), fill in Table 4-4.

Table 4-4. **Finding shorter words**

Long word	Real world or abstract?	Shorter words that mean about the same thing
herniations	real world	hernia, herniated, slipped disk, protrude, stick out
avoidance	abstract?	avoid, do not do, stay away from, quit, stop
inactivity	real world	not active, not moving, still, rest
debilitation	real world	debility, disable, loss of movement, weak, weakness, feeble
important	abstract	crucial, needed, big issue, must, matters
encouraged	abstract	allow, let, urge, suggest, try to get, ask, help
ability	abstract?	able, can, skill, power
comfortably	real world	comfort, relaxed, without pain, with little pain, ease

Long word	Real world or abstract?	Shorter words that mean about the same thing
improvement	real world?	improve, progress, doing better, doing well
condition	real world	progress, status, health, how well
exercise	real world	active, move, movement, sport
undertaken	real world	done, began, started, try
evidence	abstract	data, proof, fact
participated	real world	take part, do, join
supervised (exercise)	real world	watch, look at, manage, observe, official, program, advice, coach, plan
reduction (in pain)	real world	reduce, less, cut, feel better
benefit	abstract	help, aid, do, good
disability	real world	disable, loss of ability, debility

e. Look at the long words listed in Table 4-4. Do any of them have the same or a similar meaning?
   - *Inactivity, debilitation, and disability*
   - *Undertaken and participated*
f. Fill in Table 4-5 by listing each long word that is a nominalization and giving the root verb or adjective.

Table 4-5. **Find the root verb or adjective for each nominalization**

Nominalization	Root verb or adjective
herniations	to herniate
avoidance	to avoid
inactivity	to (not) act, inactive
debilitation	to debilitate, (dis) able
ability	able
improvement	to improve
exercise	to exercise, to exert
reduction	to reduce
benefit	to benefit
disability	to disable, (not) able

g. Does the excerpt use any compound word(s) whose meaning or pronunciation might be clearer if hyphenated or written as an open compound? If so, tell which one(s) and why you think so.
    No.

5. Looking at meaning and logic

a. What is the issue or problem this excerpt deals with?
    Patients recovering from an acute herniated disk need to stay active to keep from becoming weak.
b. With regard to this issue or problem, does the excerpt: describe it? tell why it's important? offer a solution?
    It does all three.
c. Does the excerpt frame the issue or problem in real-world terms or abstract terms? Or does it only imply the issue or problem?
    This excerpt generally describes the real world (i.e., patients recovering) but it uses many abstract-sounding terms (e.g., herniations, inactivity, debilitation, ability, improvement, benefit, disability).

C. Prescription for revising

Write your prescription for revising to treat the symptoms of *medicus incomprehensibilis*. List the things you would recommend to help improve reading ease and clarity.

- *Keep sentence length 15 words average, 25 words maximum*
- *Minimize forms of* to be
- *Revise passive into active voice*
- *Revise abstract into concrete*
- *Observe the 1066 principle*
- *Keep the subject and verb close together in the first 7 or 8 words*
- *Write in the singular*
- *Talk in terms of one doctor treating one patient*
- *Avoid using a high percentage of long words*
- *Keep essential scientific terms; minimize other long words*
- *Prefer the short word to describe the real world*
- *Convert nominalization into a verb in active voice*
- *Introduce and develop one idea in each paragraph*

D. Revision

Revise the excerpt to improve reading ease and clarity.

> It is *important* for a patient with an acute *herniated* disk to keep active, as best they can. *Otherwise*, they could become weak. A doctor should try to get the patient to stand and walk. If the patient can sit *comfortably*, it's a good sign they're improving and suggests they can try more structured *exercise*.
>
> *Evidence* of the effect of *physical therapy* and *exercise* is limited. A *systematic* review of five *randomized* trials showed that a patient in *supervised exercise* had a greater chance of short-term pain relief than one who just received counseling. But the decrease in pain was small. Over the long term, they had no less pain and no better function.

1. Looking at WSEG scores

Compute the WSEG score for your revision. Fill in Table 4-6 to show how your revision compares with the original.

Table 4-6. **Comparing WSEG scores**

WSEG		*Original*	*Revised*	*Change*
W	Number of words	109	114	5
S	Average sentence length	21.8	14.2	−7.6
E	Flesch Reading Ease score	29.4	65.4	36.0
G	Flesch-Kincaid Grade Level	14.5	7.6	−6.9

2. Looking at grammar

Answer the following questions about your revision:

a. Does each sentence put the subject and verb close together within the first 7 or 8 words? If not, tell why it seemed best to do otherwise.
   No. In paragraph 2, first sentence, the subject, "evidence," and verb, "is limited," are separated by a description of the evidence.
b. Does each sentence use active voice? If not, tell why it seemed best to do otherwise.
   No. In paragraph 1, the first and fourth sentences are neither active nor passive. In paragraph 2, the first and third sentences are neither active nor passive. We did this to track the logic of the original.

c. Does each sentence use a concrete subject? If not, tell why it seemed best to use an abstract subject.

- *Paragraph 1, first and fourth sentences—The subjects in the original were abstract; we paraphrased in more conversational language, but the paraphrase is still abstract.*
- *Paragraph 2, first, second, and third sentences—We kept the abstract subjects from the original.*

3. Prefer the short word

a. Underline each <u>long word</u>. Count the number of <u>long words</u> and compute long words as a percent of total words. <u>13</u> long words/<u>114</u> total words = <u>11.4</u>%. Compare your answer with the percent of long words in the original. (See §B.4.b.)

b. Double underline any <u>long word</u> you consider a <u>proper name</u> or <u>essential scientific term</u>.

Note

1. Plain English Campaign, "How to Write in Plain English," under "Use words that are appropriate for the reader," http://www.plainenglish.co.uk/files/howto.pdf (accessed February 1, 2018).

5

Effects of Testosterone in Older Men

Use short sentences. A good average sentence length is 15 to 20 words. Use shorter ones for 'punch'. Longer ones should not have more than three items of information; otherwise, they get overloaded, and readers lose track. —Plain English Campaign (UK), *How to Write Medical Information in Plain English*[1]

A. The excerpt

This case study looks at an excerpt from an article published in *The New England Journal of Medicine*.[2] Read the excerpt out loud:

> Seven men in each study group were adjudicated to have had major cardiovascular events (myocardial infarction, stroke, or death from cardiovascular causes) during the treatment period and two men in the testosterone group and nine men in the placebo group were adjudicated to have had major cardiovascular events during the subsequent year (Table 4, and Table S4 in the Supplementary Appendix). There was no pattern of difference in risk with respect to the other cardiovascular adverse events (Table S4 in the Supplementary Appendix). No significant between-group differences were observed in cardiac adverse events defined according to *Medical Dictionary for Regulatory Activities* classification (Tables S5 and S6 in the Supplementary Appendix). (*WSEG = 110/36.6/0.0/22.5*)

Note: The reference to "Table S4 in the Supplementary Appendix" reflects *The New England Journal of Medicine* style.

B. Analyzing the excerpt
1. Initial thoughts

What are some of your initial thoughts on this excerpt?

2. Looking at the WSEG score

a. How does this excerpt's average sentence length compare with the recommended average of 15 words?

b. How many words does each sentence use? First ____, second ____, third ____.

c. For each sentence that uses more than 25 words, do you think it needs to be just one long sentence? Why or why not?

d. Does the reading ease score fall between 45 and 70 (the one standard deviation range)? ____; or between 33 and 83 (the two standard deviation range)? ____

e. Does the grade level fall between 6 and 11 (the one standard deviation range)? ____; or between 4 and 13 (the two standard deviation range)? ____

3. Looking at grammar

a. For each sentence in the excerpt, underline the <u>subject</u> and double underline the <u>main verb</u>. If the main verb includes a past participle, then draw braces around the {<u>past participle</u>}.

b. Fill in Table 5-1, answering the questions for each sentence.

Table 5-1. **Analyze the grammar of each sentence**

Sentence	Does the main verb contain a form of *to be*?	Is the sentence active, passive or neither?	Is the subject abstract or concrete?	Are the subject and verb close together in the first 7–8 words?
1st				
2nd				
3rd				

c. For each abstract subject, explain, in your own words, why it is abstract.

d. What words or ideas are written in the plural?

e. What words or ideas need to be plural?

f. Fill in Table 5-2 to show your thinking about any phrase that shows possession or connection using *of* or a word ending other than 's.

Table 5-2. **Revising phrases that show possession or connection using *of* or a word ending**

List the phrase, underlining <u>of</u> or the <u>word ending</u>	Is the possession or connection real world or abstract?	How might you replace *of* or the word ending?

4. Prefer the short word

a. Here is a fresh copy of the excerpt. Underline each <u>long word</u>.

> Seven men in each study group were adjudicated to have had major cardiovascular events (myocardial infarction, stroke, or death from cardiovascular causes) during the treatment period and two men in the testosterone group and nine men in the placebo group were adjudicated to have had major cardiovascular events during the subsequent year (Table 4, and Table S4 in the Supplementary Appendix). There was no pattern of difference in risk with respect to the other cardiovascular adverse events (Table S4 in the Supplementary Appendix). No significant between-group differences were observed in cardiac adverse events defined according to *Medical Dictionary for Regulatory Activities* classification (Tables S5 and S6 in the Supplementary Appendix).

b. Count the number of <u>long words</u> and compute long words as a percent of total words.
   ___ long words/110 total words = ___ %

c. Double underline any <u>long word</u> you consider a <u>proper name</u> or <u>essential scientific term</u>.

d. For each <u>long word</u> you underlined just once (i.e., skip the essential scientific terms), fill in Table 5-3.

Table 5-3. **Finding shorter words**

Long word	Real world or abstract?	Shorter words that mean about the same thing

Long word	Real world or abstract?	Shorter words that mean about the same thing

e. Look at the long words listed in Table 5-3. Do any of them have the same or a similar meaning?

f. Fill in Table 5-4 by listing each long word that is a nominalization and giving the root verb or adjective.

Table 5-4. **Find the root verb or adjective for each nominalization**

Nominalization	Root verb or adjective

g. Does the excerpt use any compound word(s) whose meaning or pronunciation might be clearer if hyphenated or written as an open compound? If so, tell which one(s) and why you think so.

5. Looking at meaning and logic

a. What is the issue or problem this excerpt deals with?

b. With regard to this issue or problem, does the excerpt: describe it? tell why it is important? offer a solution?

c. Does the excerpt frame the issue or problem in real-world terms or abstract terms? Or does it only imply the issue or problem?

C. Prescription for revising

Write your prescription for revising to treat the symptoms of *medicus incomprehensibilis*. List the things you would recommend to help improve reading ease and clarity.

D. Revision

Revise the excerpt to improve reading ease and clarity.

1. Looking at WSEG scores

Compute the WSEG score for your revision. Fill in Table 5-5 to show how your revision compares with the original.

Table 5-5. **Comparing WSEG scores**

WSEG		Original	Revised	Change
W	Number of words	110		
S	Average sentence length	36.6		
E	Flesch Reading Ease score	0.0		
G	Flesch-Kincaid Grade Level	22.5		

2. Looking at grammar

Answer the following questions about your revision:

a. Does each sentence put the subject and verb close together within the first 7 or 8 words? If not, tell why it seemed best to do otherwise.

b. Does each sentence use active voice? If not, tell why it seemed best to do otherwise.

c. Does each sentence use a concrete subject? If not, tell why it seemed best to use an abstract subject.

3. Prefer the short word

a. Underline each <u>long word</u>. Count the number of <u>long words</u> and compute long words as a percent of total words. ___ long words / ___ total words = ___ %. Compare your answer with the percent of long words in the original. (See §B.4.b.)

b. Double underline any <u>long word</u> you consider a <u>proper name</u> or <u>essential scientific term</u>.

Notes

1. Plain English Campaign, "How to Write Medical Information in Plain English," under "Ten tips for clearer writing," http://www.plainenglish.co.uk/files/medicalguide.pdf (accessed January 2, 2018).
2. Peter J. Snyder, et al. "Effects of Testosterone in Older Men," *N Engl J Med* 374, no. 7 (2016): 616, 622.

Effects of Testosterone in Older Men

Using simpler words and phrases is rewarding for the reader, and for you, because it makes your writing easier to read. I could have said, "render," instead of "make," in the last sentence, but render has two syllables, so why use it? —Alistair Reeves, Time to Make It Shorter: Plain English in Our Context[1]

A. The excerpt

This case study looks at an excerpt from an article published in *The New England Journal of Medicine*. Read the excerpt out loud:

> Seven <u>men</u> in each study group <u>were {adjudicated}</u> to have had major cardiovascular events (myocardial infarction, stroke, or death from cardiovascular causes) during the treatment period and two men in the testosterone group and nine men in the placebo group were adjudicated to have had major cardiovascular events during the subsequent year (Table 4, and Table S4 in the Supplementary Appendix). <u>There was</u> no pattern of difference in risk with respect to the other cardiovascular adverse events (Table S4 in the Supplementary Appendix). No significant between-group <u>differences were {observed}</u> in cardiac adverse events defined according to *Medical Dictionary for Regulatory Activities* classification (Tables S5 and S6 in the Supplementary Appendix). (WSEG = *110/36.6/0.0/22.5*)

Note: The reference to "Table S4 in the Supplementary Appendix" reflects *The New England Journal of Medicine* style.

B. Analyzing the excerpt

1. Initial thoughts

What are some of your initial thoughts on this excerpt?
- *The first sentence is very long.*
- *"Adjudicated" is a legal term and most doctors won't know exactly what it means. They would know it means something like "judged."*
- *The excerpt uses elegant variation: cardiovascular events, cardiovascular adverse events, cardiac adverse events.*

2. Looking at the WSEG score

a. How does this excerpt's average sentence length compare with the recommended average of 15 words?
The average sentence length is 36.7 words, which is more than twice the recommended average.

b. How many words does each sentence use? First <u>61</u>, second <u>22</u>, third <u>27</u>

c. For each sentence that uses more than 25 words, do you think it needs to be just one long sentence? Why or why not?

   - *The first sentence, which uses 61 words, could be broken up. We could say, in one sentence, that seven men in each group were judged to have had major cardiovascular events during the treatment period. In another sentence, we could say what those major cardiovascular events were. In yet another sentence, we could say that two men in the testosterone group and nine men in the placebo group were adjudicated to have had major cardiovascular events in the following year. Then, in still another sentence, we could refer the reader to Table 4, and Table S4 in the Supplementary Appendix.*

   - *The third sentence, which uses 27 words, could be broken up into two sentences. We could say, in one sentence, no significant between-group differences were observed in cardiac adverse events, as defined by the* Medical Dictionary for Regulatory Activities. *Then, in another sentence, we could refer the reader to Table S5 and S6 in the Supplementary Appendix.*

d. Does the reading ease score fall between 45 and 70 (the one standard deviation range)? <u>*No*</u>; or between 33 and 83 (the two standard deviation range)? <u>*No*</u>

e. Does the grade level fall between 6 and 11 (the one standard deviation range)? <u>*No*</u>; or between 4 and 13 (the two standard deviation range)? <u>*No*</u>

3. Looking at grammar

a. For each sentence in the excerpt, underline the <u>subject</u> and double underline the <u>main verb</u>. If the main verb includes a past participle, then draw braces around the {<u>past participle</u>}.

b. Fill in Table 5-1, answering the questions for each sentence.

Table 5-1. **Analyze the grammar of each sentence**

Sentence	Does the main verb contain a form of to be?	Is the sentence active, passive or neither?	Is the subject abstract or concrete?	Are the subject and verb close together in the first 7–8 words?
1st	yes	passive	concrete	yes
2nd	yes	neither	abstract	yes
3rd	yes	passive	abstract	yes

c. For each abstract subject, explain, in your own words, why it is abstract.
  *   *"There" stands in place of "pattern of difference of risk," which is abstract because it involves a conclusion based on analysis.*
  *   *"(Between-group) differences" involves analysis.*

d. What words or ideas are written in the plural?
  Men, events, causes, differences, Activities, Tables

e. What words or ideas need to be plural?
  Men, events, causes, Activities, Tables

f. Fill in Table 5-2 to show your thinking about any phrase that shows possession or connection using *of* or a word ending other than 's.

Table 5-2. **Revising phrases that show possession or connection using *of*** **or a word ending**

List the phrase, underlining of or the word ending	Is the possession or connection real world or abstract?	How might you replace of or the word ending?
major cardiovascul<u>ar</u> events	real world	major heart or blood vessel events
myocardi<u>al</u> infarction	real world	heart attack
cardiovascul<u>ar</u> causes	real world	heart or blood vessel causes
pattern <u>of</u> difference	abstract	(no change)
cardiovascul<u>ar</u> adverse events	real world	heart or blood vessel adverse events
cardi<u>ac</u> adverse events	real world	heart adverse events

4. Prefer the short word

a. Here is a fresh copy of the excerpt. Underline each <u>long word</u>.

> Seven men in each study group were <u>adjudicated</u> to have had major <u>cardiovascular</u> events (<u>myocardial</u> <u>infarction</u>, stroke, or death from <u>cardiovascular</u> causes) during the treatment <u>period</u> and two men in the <u>testosterone</u> group and nine men in the <u>placebo</u> group were <u>adjudicated</u> to have had major <u>cardiovascular</u> events during the <u>subsequent</u> year (Table 4, and Table S4 in the <u>Supplementary</u> <u>Appendix</u>). There was no pattern of <u>difference</u> in risk with respect to the other <u>cardiovascular</u> adverse events (Table S4 in the <u>Supplementary</u> <u>Appendix</u>). No <u>significant</u> <u>between-group</u> <u>differences</u> were observed in <u>cardiac</u> adverse events defined according to <u>Medical</u> <u>Dictionary</u> <u>for</u> <u>Regulatory</u> <u>Activities</u> <u>classification</u> (Tables S5 and S6 in the <u>Supplementary</u> <u>Appendix</u>).

b. Count the number of <u>long words</u> and compute long words as a percent of total words.
   <u>28</u> long words/110 total words = <u>25.5</u>%

c. Double underline any <u>long word</u> you consider a <u>proper name</u> or <u>essential scientific term</u>.

d. For each <u>long word</u> you underlined just once (i.e., skip the essential scientific terms), fill in Table 5-3.

Table 5-3. **Finding shorter words**

Long word	Real world or abstract?	Shorter words that mean about the same thing
adjudicated	abstract	judge, examine, decide, determine, found
cardiovascular	real world	heart and blood vessels
myocardial	real world	heart, heart tissue, heart muscle, cardiac
infarction	real world	tissue death, muscle death, (heart) attack
period	abstract	time, span, phase, stage, during
subsequent	abstract	next, after, later, following
difference	abstract	differ, gap, not same, change, unlike, not like
significant	abstract	notable, important, big, large, major
between-group	abstract	two or more groups, between the two groups

Long word	Real world or abstract?	Shorter words that mean about the same thing
cardiac	real world	heart
classification	abstract	classify, definition, define, list

e. Look at the long words listed in Table 5-3. Do any of them have the same or a similar meaning?
   • *Adjudicated and classification*
   • *Cardiovascular, myocardial and cardiac*
   • *Difference and between-group*
f. Fill in Table 5-4 by listing each long word that is a nominalization and giving the root verb or adjective.

Table 5-4. **Find the root verb or adjective for each nominalization**

Nominalization	Root verb or adjective
infarction	to infarct
difference	to differ
classification	to classify

g. Does the excerpt use any compound word(s) whose meaning or pronunciation might be clearer if hyphenated or written as an open compound? If so, tell which one(s) and why you think so.
   We might hyphenate "cardio-vascular," so the reader can better see the two parts.

5. Looking at meaning and logic

a. What is the issue or problem this excerpt deals with?
   How testosterone affects cardiovascular events in men.
b. With regard to this issue or problem, does the excerpt: describe it? tell why it is important? offer a solution?
   The excerpt deals with research methods and results for a study seeking to determine the extent of the problem. It seeks to tell if and why the problem is important. It may also help point the way to a solution.
c. Does the excerpt frame the issue or problem in real-world terms or abstract terms? Or does it only imply the issue or problem?
   In this excerpt, the problem is implied (apparently stated explicitly at the beginning of the article).

C. Prescription for revising

Write your prescription for revising to treat the symptoms of *medicus incomprehensibilis*. List the things you would recommend to help improve reading ease and clarity.
- *Keep sentence length 15 words average, 25 words maximum*
- *Revise passive into active voice*
- *Revise abstract into concrete*
- *Observe the 1066 principle*
- *Avoid using a high percentage of long words*
- *Keep essential scientific terms; minimize other long words*
- *Use terms consistently; avoid elegant variation*
- *Omit any needless word*

D. Revision

Revise the excerpt to improve reading ease and clarity.

> *Seven men in each study group were judged to have had a major heart or blood vessel event during the treatment period. These events included heart attack, stroke, or death from heart or blood vessel causes. Two men in the testosterone group and nine in the placebo group were judged to have had a major heart or blood vessel event in the next year. (See Table 4, and Table S4 in the Supplementary Appendix.)*
>
> *We saw no pattern of difference in risk with respect to the other heart or blood vessel adverse events. (See Table S4 in the Supplementary Appendix.) We also saw no difference between the groups in heart adverse events as defined in the Medical Dictionary for Regulatory Activities. (See Tables S5 and S6 in the Supplementary Appendix.)*

1. Looking at WSEG scores

Compute the WSEG score for your revision. Fill in Table 5-5 to show how your revision compares with the original.

Table 5-5. **Comparing WSEG scores**

WSEG		Original	Revised	Change
W	Number of words	110	129	19
S	Average sentence length	36.6	16.1	−20.5
E	Flesch Reading Ease score	0.0	58.6	58.6
G	Flesch-Kincaid Grade Level	22.5	9.0	−13.5

2. Looking at grammar

Answer the following questions about your revision:

a. Does each sentence put the subject and verb close together within the first 7 or 8 words? If not, tell why it seemed best to do otherwise.
   No. In paragraph 1, third sentence, the long logical subject keeps us from putting the grammatical subject, "men," and verb, "were judged," together in the first 7 or 8 words.

b. Does each sentence use active voice? If not, tell why it seemed best to do otherwise.
   No. Paragraph 1, the first and third sentences are passive. What was judged is important, but who did the judging is not.

c. Does each sentence use a concrete subject? If not, tell why it seemed best to use an abstract subject.
   Yes. Each sentence uses a concrete subject.

3. Prefer the short word

a. Underline each <u>long word</u>. Count the number of <u>long words</u> and compute long words as a percent of total words. <u>15</u> long words/<u>129</u> total words = <u>11.6</u>%. Compare your answer with the percent of long words in the original. (See §B.4.b.)

b. Double underline any <u>long word</u> you consider a <u>proper name</u> or <u>essential scientific term</u>.

Note

1. Alistair Reeves, "Time to Make It Shorter: Plain English in Our Context," *Medical Writing* 24, no. 1 (2015): 8.

Atrial Fibrillation and the Risk of Heart, Blood Vessel, and Kidney Disease

The process of linguistic change is inevitable, and grammatical rigor must be tempered by judgment and common sense. —The AMA Manual of Style[1]

A. The excerpt

This case study looks at an excerpt from an article published in *The BMJ (British Medical Journal).*[2] Read the excerpt out loud:

> We abstracted relative risk estimates and associated 95% confidence intervals for the association between atrial fibrillation and all cause mortality, cardiovascular mortality, major cardiovascular events (a composite of cardiovascular death, fatal and non-fatal stroke, ischaemic heart disease, and congestive heart failure), and disease specific events: fatal and non-fatal stroke (all stroke or a stroke subtype if all stroke was not provided), fatal and non-fatal haemorrhagic stroke, fatal and non-fatal ischaemic stroke, ischaemic heart disease events (a composite of ischaemic heart disease death and non-fatal myocardial infarction), incident development of congestive heart failure, chronic kidney disease, and peripheral arterial disease. Maximally adjusted relative risk estimates were abstracted, along with the list of covariates included in the published multivariable regression model. Studies that did not report the variables that were adjusted for were excluded. One study that reported the development of end stage renal disease was included in the meta-analysis of chronic kidney disease. (*WSEG = 152/38.0/0.0/23.8*)

B. Analyzing the excerpt

1. Initial thoughts

What are some of your initial thoughts on this excerpt?

2. Looking at the WSEG score

a. Is the paragraph longer than 150 words? ____ If so, do you see a good way to split it into shorter paragraphs?

b. How does this excerpt's average sentence length compare with the recommended average of 15 words?

c. Count the number of words in each sentence. Then calculate the total number of words for the excerpt. Write your answers in Table 6-1.

Table 6-1. **Words per sentence**

	Sentence				
	1st	*2nd*	*3rd*	*4th*	*Total*
Number of words					

d. For each sentence that uses more than 25 words, do you think it needs to be just one long sentence? Why or why not?

e. Does the reading ease score fall between 45 and 70 (the one standard deviation range)?____; or between 33 and 83 (the two standard deviation range)? ____

f. Does the grade level fall between 6 and 11 (the one standard deviation range)? ____; or between 4 and 13 (the two standard deviation range)? ____

3. Looking at grammar

a. For each sentence in the excerpt, underline the <u>subject</u> and double underline the <u>main verb</u>. If the main verb includes a past participle, then draw
braces around the {<u>past participle</u>}.

b. Fill in Table 6-2, answering the questions for each sentence.

Table 6-2. **Analyze the grammar of each sentence**

Sentence	*Does the main verb contain a form of* to be?	*Is the sentence active, passive or neither?*	*Is the subject abstract or concrete?*	*Are the subject and verb close together in the first 7–8 words?*
1st				
2nd				
3rd				
4th				

c. For each abstract subject, explain, in your own words, why it is abstract.

d. What words or ideas are written in the plural?

e. What words or ideas need to be plural?

f. Fill in Table 6-3 to show your thinking about any phrase that shows
possession or connection using *of* or a word ending other than *'s*.

Table 6-3. **Revising phrases that show possession or connection using** *of*
                or a word ending

List the phrase, underlining <u>of</u> *or the* <u>word ending</u>	*Is the possession or connection real world or abstract?*	*How might you replace* of *or the word ending?*

List the phrase, underlining <u>of</u> or the <u>word</u> ending	*Is the possession or connection real world or abstract?*	*How might you replace of or the word ending?*

4. Prefer the short word

a. Here is a fresh copy of the excerpt. Underline each <u>long word.</u>

We abstracted relative risk estimates and associated 95% confidence intervals for the association between atrial fibrillation and all cause mortality, cardiovascular mortality, major cardiovascular events (a composite of cardiovascular death, fatal and non-fatal stroke, ischaemic heart disease, and congestive heart failure), and disease specific events: fatal and non-fatal stroke (all stroke or a stroke subtype if all stroke was not provided), fatal and non-fatal haemorrhagic stroke, fatal and non-fatal ischaemic stroke, ischaemic heart disease events (a composite of ischaemic heart disease death and non-fatal myocardial infarction), incident development of congestive heart failure, chronic kidney disease, and peripheral arterial disease. Maximally adjusted relative risk estimates were abstracted, along with the list of covariates included in the published multivariable regression model. Studies that did not report the variables that were adjusted for were excluded. One study that reported the development of end stage renal disease was included in the meta-analysis of chronic kidney disease.

b. Count the number of <u>long words</u> and compute long words as a percent of total words.

___ long words/152 total words = ___ %

c. Double underline any <u>long word</u> you consider a <u>proper name</u> or <u>essential scientific term</u>.

d. For each <u>long word</u> you underlined just once (i.e., skip the essential scientific terms), fill in Table 6-4.

Table 6-4. **Finding shorter words**

Long word	Real world or abstract?	Shorter words that mean about the same thing

e. Look at the long words listed in Table 6-4. Do any of them have the same or a similar meaning?

f. Fill in Table 6-5 by listing each long word that is a nominalization and giving the root verb or adjective.

Table 6-5. **Find the root verb or adjective for each nominalization**

Nominalization	Root verb or adjective

g. Does the excerpt use any compound word(s) whose meaning or pronunciation might be clearer if hyphenated or written as an open compound? If so, tell which one(s) and why you think so.

5. Looking at meaning and logic

a. Here is a fresh copy of the excerpt. Re-read the excerpt and strike out any word you think is not needed to understand the excerpt's main idea. Do minor re-arranging or editing, if needed.

> We abstracted relative risk estimates and associated 95% confidence intervals for the association between atrial fibrillation and all cause mortality, cardiovascular mortality, major cardiovascular death events (a composite of cardiovascular, fatal and non-fatal stroke, ischaemic heart disease, and congestive heart failure), and disease specific events: fatal and non-fatal stroke (all stroke or a stroke subtype if all stroke was not provided), fatal and non-fatal haemorrhagic stroke, fatal and non-fatal ischaemic stroke, ischaemic heart disease events (a composite of ischaemic heart disease death and non-fatal myocardial infarction), incident development of congestive heart failure, chronic kidney disease, and peripheral arterial disease. Maximally adjusted relative risk estimates were abstracted, along with the list of covariates included in the published multivariable

regression model. Studies that did not report the variables that were adjusted for were excluded. One study that reported the development of end stage renal disease was included in the meta-analysis of chronic kidney disease.

b. What is the issue or problem this excerpt deals with?

c. With regard to this issue or problem, does the excerpt: describe it? tell why it is important? offer a solution?

d. Does the excerpt frame the issue or problem in real-world terms or abstract terms? Or does it only imply the issue or problem?

C. Prescription for revising

Write your prescription for revising to treat the symptoms of *medicus incomprehensibilis*. List the things you would recommend to help improve reading ease and clarity.

D. Revision

Revise the excerpt to improve reading ease and clarity.

1. Looking at WSEG scores

Compute the WSEG score for your revision. Fill in Table 6-6 to show how your revision compares with the original.

Table 6-6. **Comparing WSEG scores**

WSEG		Original	Revised	Change
W	Number of words	152		
S	Average sentence length	38.0		
E	Flesch Reading Ease score	0.0		
G	Flesch-Kincaid Grade Level	23.8		

2. Looking at grammar

Answer the following questions about your revision:

a. Does each sentence put the subject and verb close together within the first 7 or 8 words? If not, tell why it seemed best to do otherwise.

b. Does each sentence use active voice? If not, tell why it seemed best to do otherwise.

c. Does each sentence use a concrete subject? If not, tell why it seemed best to use an abstract subject.

3. Prefer the short word

a. Underline each long word. Count the number of long words and compute long words as a percent of total words. ___ long words/___ total words = ___ %. Compare your answer with the percent of long words in the original. (See §B.4.b.)

b. Double underline any long word you consider a proper name or essential scientific term.

Notes

1. Cheryl Iverson et al., *The AMA Manual of Style: A Guide for Authors and Editors*, 10th ed. (Oxford, UK: Oxford University Press, 2007), sec. 7.1.1.
2. Ayodele Odutayo, et al., "Atrial Fibrillation and Risk of Cardiovascular Disease, Renal Disease, and Death: Systematic Review and Meta-analysis," *BMJ* 354, no. 8072 (September 6, 2016), under "Data Extraction and Quality Assessment," https://www.bmj.com/content/354/bmj.i4482.

Atrial Fibrillation and the Risk of Heart, Blood Vessel, and Kidney Disease

It does no harm to challenge producers of over-complex writing, whoever they may be. —Martin Cutts[1]

A. The excerpt

This case study looks at an excerpt from an article published in *The BMJ (British Medical Journal)*. Read the excerpt out loud:

> We <u>abstracted</u> relative risk estimates and associated 95% confidence intervals for the association between atrial fibrillation and all cause mortality, cardiovascular mortality, major cardiovascular events (a composite of cardiovascular death, fatal and non-fatal stroke, ischaemic heart disease, and congestive heart failure), and disease specific events: fatal and non-fatal stroke (all stroke or a stroke subtype if all stroke was not provided), fatal and non-fatal haemorrhagic stroke, fatal and non-fatal ischaemic stroke, ischaemic heart disease events (a composite of ischaemic heart disease death and non-fatal myocardial infarction), incident development of congestive heart failure, chronic kidney disease, and peripheral arterial disease. Maximally adjusted relative risk <u>estimates</u> <u>were {abstracted}</u>, along with the list of covariates included in the published multivariable regression model. <u>Studies</u> that did not report the variables that were adjusted for <u>were {excluded}</u>. One <u>study</u> that reported the development of end stage renal disease <u>was {included}</u> in the meta-analysis of chronic kidney disease. (*WSEG = 152/38.0/0.0/23.8*)

B. Analyzing the excerpt
1. Initial thoughts

What are some of your initial thoughts on this excerpt?
- *The first sentence is way too long! It has a list, with sub-lists and sub-sub-lists.*
- *The paragraph is a little long.*
- *It uses many medical terms.*

2. Looking at the WSEG score

a. Is the paragraph longer than 150 words? <u>*Yes*</u>. If so, do you see a good way to split it into shorter paragraphs?
   We could split it into two paragraphs. In one paragraph, we could talk about what we (i.e., the researchers) did. Then, in another paragraph, we could give details about how we did it.

b. How does this excerpt's average sentence length compare with the recommended average of 15 words?
   It has an average sentence length of 38.0 words—more than 2.5 times the recommended average.

c. Count the number of words in each sentence. Then calculate the total number of words for the excerpt. Write your answers in Table 6-1.

Table 6-1. **Words per sentence**

	Sentence				
	1st	*2nd*	*3rd*	*4th*	*Total*
Number of words	*99*	*20*	*13*	*20*	*152*

d. For each sentence that uses more than 25 words, do you think it needs to be just one long sentence? Why or why not?
   The first sentence, which uses 99 words, could be broken up into several sentences. We could say, in one sentence, we looked at how atrial fibrillation is associated with death from all causes and a wide range of cardiovascular events. Then, in another sentence, we could say, we abstracted relative risk estimates for these associations and their 95% confidence intervals. Then, in yet another sentence, we could say what we included as major cardiovascular events. Then, in still another sentence, we could say what we included as disease specific events.

e. Does the reading ease score fall between 45 and 70 (the one standard deviation range)? <u>*No*</u>; or between 33 and 83 (the two standard deviation range)? <u>*No*</u>

f. Does the grade level fall between 6 and 11 (the one standard deviation range)? <u>*No*</u>; or between 4 and 13 (the two standard deviation range)? <u>*No*</u>

3. Looking at grammar

a. For each sentence in the excerpt, underline the <u>subject</u> and double under-line the <u>main verb</u>. If the main verb includes a past participle, then draw braces around the {<u>past participle</u>}.

b. Fill in Table 6-2, answering the questions for each sentence.

Table 6-2. **Analyze the grammar of each sentence**

Sentence	*Does the main verb contain a form of* to be?	*Is the sentence active, passive or neither?*	*Is the subject abstract or concrete?*	*Are the subject and verb close together in the first 7–8 words?*
1st	no	active	concrete	yes
2nd	yes	passive	abstract	yes
3rd	yes	passive	abstract	no
4th	yes	passive	abstract	no

c. For each abstract subject, explain, in your own words, why it is abstract.
   • *"Estimates" involves analysis or a statistical calculation.*
   • *"Studies/study" involves real-world actions guided by abstract thought and analysis.*

d. What words or ideas are written in the plural?
   Estimates, intervals, events, covariates, studies, variables

e. What words or ideas need to be plural?
   Events, covariates, studies, variables

f. Fill in Table 6-3 to show your thinking about any phrase that shows possession or connection using *of* or a word ending other than *'s.*

Table 6-3. **Revising phrases that show possession or connection using *of* or a word ending**

List the phrase, underlining <u>of</u> or the word <u>ending</u>	Is the possession or connection real world or abstract?	How might you replace of or the word ending?
atri<u>al</u> fibrillation	real world	*(no change—essential scientific term)*
cardiovascul<u>ar</u> mortality	real world	*death (rates) from heart and blood vessel causes*
cardiovascul<u>ar</u> events	real world	*heart and blood vessel events*
composite <u>of</u> . . .	abstract	*including . . .*

List the phrase, underlining <u>of</u> or the word <u>ending</u>	Is the possession or connection real world or abstract?	How might you replace of or the word ending?
cardiovascul<u>ar</u> death	real world	death from heart and blood vessel causes
ischaem<u>ic</u> heart disease	real world	(no change)
haemorrhag<u>ic</u> stroke	real world	stroke caused by bleeding in the brain
ischaem<u>ic</u> stroke	real world	(no change)
myocard<u>ial</u> infarction	real world	heart attack
incident develop<u>ment</u> <u>of</u> congestive heart failure	real world	congestive heart failure
chro<u>nic</u> kidney disease	real world	(no change)
periphe<u>ral</u> arte<u>rial</u> disease	real world	periphe<u>ral</u> artery disease
list <u>of</u> covariates	abstract	(no change)
study that reported on the development <u>of</u> end stage ren<u>al</u> disease	study—abstract; end stage renal disease—real world	study on end stage kidney disease
meta-analy<u>sis</u> <u>of</u> chro<u>nic</u> kidney diseases	abstract	(no change)

4. Prefer the short word

a. Here is a fresh copy of the excerpt. Underline each <u>long word.</u>

> We abstracted <u>relative</u> risk <u>estimates</u> and <u>associated</u> 95% <u>confidence</u> <u>intervals</u> for the <u>association</u> between <u>atrial</u> <u>fibrillation</u> and all cause <u>mortality</u>, <u>cardiovascular</u> <u>mortality</u>, major <u>cardiovascular</u> events (a <u>composite</u> of <u>cardiovascular</u> death, fatal and <u>non-fatal</u> stroke, <u>ischaemic</u> heart disease, and <u>congestive</u> heart failure), and disease <u>specific</u> events: fatal and <u>non-fatal</u> stroke (all stroke or a stroke subtype if all stroke was not provided), fatal and <u>non-fatal</u> <u>haemorrhagic</u> stroke, fatal and <u>non-fatal</u> <u>ischaemic</u> stroke, <u>ischaemic</u> heart disease events (a <u>composite</u> of <u>ischaemic</u> heart disease death and <u>non-fatal</u> <u>myocardial</u> <u>infarction</u>), <u>incident</u> <u>development</u> of <u>congestive</u> heart failure, chronic kidney disease, and <u>peripheral</u> <u>arterial</u> disease. <u>Maximally</u> adjusted <u>relative</u> risk <u>estimates</u> were abstracted, along with the list of <u>covariates</u> included in the published <u>multivariable</u> <u>regression</u> model. Studies that did not report the <u>variables</u> that were adjusted for were excluded. One

study that reported the <u>development</u> of end stage renal disease
was included in the <u>meta-analysis</u> of chronic kidney disease.

b. Count the number of <u>long words</u> and compute long words as a percent of
total words.

<u>43</u> long words/152 total words = <u>28.3</u>%

c. Double underline any <u>long word</u> you consider a <u>proper name</u> or <u>essential
scientific term</u>.

d. For each <u>long word</u> you underlined just once (i.e., skip the essential scientific terms), fill in Table 6-4.

Table 6-4. **Finding shorter words**

Long word	Real world or abstract?	Shorter words that mean about the same thing
relative	abstract	related, compare, (risk) ratio
estimates	abstract	guess, predicted, likely, expect, number, ratio
associated	abstract	related, connected, linked, paired, also
association	abstract	connection, cause, pairing, relate, relation, relationship, link
mortality	real world	death, death rate, number of deaths, mortal
cardiovascular	real world	heart and blood vessels
composite	abstract	compose, mix, blend, including, meaning, e.g., arrange
non-fatal	real world	not fatal, will not kill
ischemic	real world	restricted blood flow, block, blockage, clot
congestive	real world	congest, excess blood, clog, block
specific	abstract	unique, only, just for
haemorrhagic	real world	bleeding, blood vessel rupture
myocardial	real world	heart, heart tissue, heart muscle, cardiac
infarction	real world	infarct, tissue death, muscle death, (heart) attack
incident	abstract	event, harmful event
development	abstract	develop
arterial	real world	artery, blood vessels
maximally	abstract	maximum, maximal, as much as possible, highest, optimize, most

e. Look at the long words listed in Table 6-4. Do any of them have the same or a similar meaning?
- *Associated and associations*
- *Cardiovascular and arterial*

f. Fill in Table 6-5 by listing each long word that is a nominalization and giving the root verb or adjective.

Table 6-5. **Find the root verb or adjective for each nominalization**

Nominalization	Root verb or adjective
estimates	*to estimate*
association	*to associate*
mortality	*mortal*
composite	*to compose*
infarction	*to infarct*
development	*to develop*

g. Does the excerpt use any compound word(s) whose meaning or pronunciation might be clearer if hyphenated or written as an open compound? If so, tell which one(s) and why you think so.
We might hyphenate "cardio-vascular," "multi-variable," and "co-variate" so people can better see the two parts.

5. Looking at meaning and logic

a. Here is a fresh copy of the excerpt. Re-read the excerpt and strike out any word you think is not needed to understand the excerpt's main idea. Do minor re-arranging or editing, if needed.

> We abstracted relative risk estimates and ~~associated~~ 95% confidence intervals for the association between atrial fibrillation and all cause mortality, cardiovascular mortality, major cardiovascular death ~~events (a composite of cardiovascular, fatal and non-fatal stroke, ischaemic heart disease, and congestive heart failure)~~, and disease specific events: fatal and non-fatal stroke ~~(all stroke or a stroke subtype if all stroke was not provided), fatal and non-fatal haemorrhagic stroke, fatal and non-fatal ischaemic stroke,~~ ischaemic heart disease ~~events (a composite of ischaemic heart disease death and non-fatal myocardial infarction), incident development of~~ congestive heart failure, chronic kidney disease, and peripheral

arterial disease. Maximally adjusted relative risk estimates were abstracted, along with the list of covariates included in the published multivariable regression model. Studies that did not report the variables that were adjusted for were excluded. One study ~~that reported the development~~ of end stage renal disease was included in the meta-analysis of chronic kidney disease.

b. What is the issue or problem this excerpt deals with?
    What is the association between (1) atrial fibrillation and (2) death and other health events?
c. With regard to this issue or problem, does the excerpt: describe it? tell why it is important? offer a solution?
    It describes how the researchers did the statistical analysis.
d. Does the excerpt frame the issue or problem in real world terms or abstract terms? or does it only imply the issue or problem?
    The adverse events are real world. The statistical analysis is abstract.

C. Prescription for revising

Write your prescription for revising to treat the symptoms of *medicus incomprehensibilis*. List the things you would recommend to help improve reading ease and clarity.

- *Keep sentence length 15 words average, 25 words maximum*
- *Revise passive into active voice*
- *Revise abstract into concrete*
- *Observe the 1066 principle*
- *Keep the subject and verb close together in the first 7 or 8 words*
- *Keep essential scientific terms; minimize other long words*
- *Omit any needless word*

D. Revision

Revise the excerpt to improve reading ease and clarity.

We studied how atrial fibrillation is associated with (1) death from all causes and (2) a wide range of heart and blood vessels events. We abstracted relative risk estimates for these associations and their 95% confidence intervals.

The heart or blood vessel events included death, fatal and non-fatal stroke caused by clots or bleeding, ischaemic heart disease, and congestive heart failure. The disease specific events included fatal and non-fatal stroke, ischaemic heart disease, <u>congestive</u> heart failure, chronic kidney disease, and <u>peripheral</u> <u>artery</u> disease.

    We abstracted <u>optimized</u> <u>relative</u> risk <u>estimates</u>, and the list of <u>co-variates</u> that were part of the published <u>multi-variable</u> <u>regression</u> model. We left out any study that did not report the <u>variables</u> we adjusted for. The <u>meta-analysis</u> of chronic kidney disease included one study on end stage kidney disease.

1. Looking at WSEG scores

Compute the WSEG score for your revision. Fill in Table 6-6 to show how your revision compares with the original.

Table 6-6. **Comparing WSEG scores**

WSEG		*Original*	*Revised*	*Change*
W	Number of words	152	131	–21
S	Average sentence length	38.0	18.7	–19.3
E	Flesch Reading Ease score	0.0	35.4	35.4
G	Flesch-Kincaid Grade Level	23.8	12.9	–10.9

2. Looking at grammar

Answer the following questions about your revision:

a. Does each sentence put the subject and verb close together within the first 7 or 8 words? If not, tell why it seemed best to do otherwise.
    Yes.
b. Does each sentence use active voice? If not, tell why it seemed best to do otherwise.
    Yes.
c. Does each sentence use a concrete subject? If not, tell why it seemed best to use an abstract subject.
    Any discussion of statistical analysis is inherently abstract. Therefore, our revision kept two original abstract subjects: events and meta-analysis.

3. Prefer the short word

a. Underline each <u>long word</u>. Count the number of long words and compute long words as a percent of total words. <u>25</u> long words/<u>131</u> total words = <u>19.1</u>%. Compare your answer with the percent of long words in the original. (See §B.4.b.)

b. Double underline any <u>long word</u> you consider a <u>proper name</u> or <u>essential scientific term</u>.

Note

1. Martin Cutts, "Making Leaflets Clearer for Patients," *Medical Writing* 24, no. 1 (2015): 17.

7

Glucose Lowering Drugs in Patients with Type 2 Diabetes

Hemoglobin is the protein inside red blood cells that carries oxygen. Red blood cells also remove carbon dioxide from your body, transporting it to the lungs for you to exhale. Red blood cells are made inside your bones, in the bone marrow. They typically live for about 120 days, and then they die. —Health Encyclopedia, University of Rochester Medical Center (New York, USA)[1]

A. The excerpt

This case study looks at an excerpt from an article published in *JAMA: The Journal of the American Medical Association.*[2] Read the excerpt out loud:

> Drugs as monotherapy were associated with large proportional reductions in HbA_{1c} levels compared with placebo, while metformin was associated with moderately lower HbA_{1c} levels compared with other drugs including sulfonylureas, thiazolidinediones, and DPP-4 inhibitors. Basal insulin and sulfonylureas were associated with greatest odds of hypoglycemia, with an absolute risk difference of 10% compared with metformin. Metformin was associated with small reductions in body weight relative to sulfonylurea or thiazolidinedione treatment. Considering these results, with metformin showing favorable associations with HbA_{1c} levels compared with sulfonylureas, thiazolidinediones, and DPP-4 inhibitors, and without adverse signals for hypoglycemia or weight gain, metformin might be considered a reasonable first-line agent for type 2 diabetes, consistent with the American Diabetes Association recommendations. However, the recommendations also suggested a patient-centered approach—considering efficacy, weight gain, hypoglycemia, and comorbidities—when selecting treatment. Therefore, based on this review, clinicians and patients may prefer to avoid sulfonylureas or basal insulin for patients who wish to minimize hypoglycemia, choose GLP-1 receptor agonists when weight management is a priority, or consider SGLT-2 inhibitors based on their favorable combined safety and efficacy profile. (WSEG = 180/30.0/0.0/23.3)

Notes:

1. Metformin, insulins, sulfonylureas, thiazolidinediones, DPP-4 inhibitors, SGLT-2 inhibitors, and GLP-1 receptor agonists are glucose-lowering drug classes approved for type 2 diabetes.[3]
2. *HbA$_{1C}$* stands for *hemoglobin A$_{1c}$* or *glycated hemoglobin*. A hemoglobin molecule glycates when it binds with a glucose molecule. How many glucose molecules bind with a hemoglobin molecule depends on the total glucose in the bloodstream at the time. Since a human red blood cell lives for 8–12 weeks, checking a person's HbA$_{1c}$ level also shows their average blood glucose level over the past 8–12 weeks.[4]

B. Analyzing the excerpt

1. Initial thoughts

What are some of your initial thoughts on this excerpt?

2. Looking at the WSEG score

a. Is the paragraph longer than 150 words? ___ If so, do you see a good way to split it into shorter paragraphs?

b. How does this excerpt's average sentence length compare with the recommended average of 15 words?

c. Count the number of words in each sentence. Then calculate the total number of words. Write your answers in Table 7-1.

Table 7-1. **Words per sentence**

	Sentence						
	1st	*2nd*	*3rd*	*4th*	*5th*	*6th*	*Total*
Number of words							

d. For each sentence that uses more than 25 words, do you think it needs to be just one long sentence? Why or why not?

e. Does the reading ease score fall between 45 and 70 (the one standard deviation range)?___; or between 33 and 83 (the two standard deviation range)? ___

f. Does the grade level fall between 6 and 11 (the one standard deviation range)? ___; or between 4 and 13 (the two standard deviation range)? ___

3. Looking at grammar

a. For each sentence in the excerpt, underline the <u>subject</u> and double under-line the <u>main verb</u>. If the main verb includes a past participle, draw braces around the {<u>past participle</u>}.

b. Fill in Table 7-2, answering the questions for each sentence.

Table 7-2. **Analyze the grammar of each sentence**

Sentence	Does the main verb contain a form of to be?	Is the sentence active, passive or neither?	Is the subject abstract or concrete?	Are the subject and verb close together in the first 7–8 words?
1st				
2nd				
3rd				
4th				
5th				
6th				

c. For each abstract subject, explain, in your own words, why it is abstract.

d. What words or ideas are written in the plural?

e. What words or ideas need to be plural?

f. Fill in Table 7-3 to show your thinking about any phrase that shows possession or connection using *of* or a word ending other than '*s*.

Table 7-3. **Revising phrases that show possession or connection using *of* or a word ending**

List the phrase, underlining <u>of</u> or the <u>word ending</u>	Is the possession or connection real world or abstract?	How might you replace of or the word ending?

List the phrase, underlining <u>of</u> or the <u>word</u> <u>ending</u>	Is the possession or connection real world or abstract?	How might you replace of or the word ending?

4. Prefer the short word

a. Here is a fresh copy of the excerpt. Underline each <u>long word</u>.

> Drugs as monotherapy were associated with large proportional reductions in HbA_{1c} levels compared with placebo, while metformin was associated with moderately lower HbA_{1c} levels compared with other drugs including sulfonylureas, thiazolidinediones, and DPP-4 inhibitors. Basal insulin and sulfonylureas were associated with greatest odds of hypoglycemia, with an absolute risk difference of 10% compared with metformin. Metformin was associated with small reductions in body weight relative to sulfonylurea or thiazolidinedione treatment. Considering these results, with metformin showing favorable associations with HbA_{1c} levels compared with sulfonylureas, thiazolidinediones, and DPP-4 inhibitors, and without adverse signals for hypoglycemia or weight gain, metformin might be considered a reasonable first-line agent for type 2 diabetes, consistent with the American Diabetes Association recommendations. However, the recommendations also suggested a patient-centered approach—considering efficacy, weight gain, hypoglycemia, and comorbidities—when selecting treatment. Therefore, based on this review, clinicians and patients may prefer to avoid sulfonylureas or basal insulin for patients who wish to minimize hypoglycemia, choose GLP-1 receptor agonists when weight management is a priority, or consider SGLT-2 inhibitors based on their favorable combined safety and efficacy profile.

b. Count the number of <u>long words</u> and compute long words as a percent of total words.
    ____ long words/180 total words = ____ %.

c. Double underline any <u>long word</u> you consider a <u>proper name</u> or <u>essential scientific term</u>.

d. For each <u>long word</u> you underlined just once (i.e., skip the essential scientific terms), fill in Table 7-4.

Table 7-4. **Finding shorter words**

Long word	Real world or abstract?	Shorter words that mean about the same thing

e. Look at the long words listed in Table 7-4. Do any of them have the same or a similar meaning?

f. Fill in Table 7-5 by listing each long word that is a nominalization and giving the root verb or adjective.

Table 7-5. **Find the root verb or adjective for each nominalization**

Nominalization	Root verb or adjective

g. Does the excerpt use any compound word(s) whose meaning or pronunciation might be clearer if hyphenated or written as an open compound? If so, tell which one(s) and why you think so.

5. Looking at meaning and logic

a. What is the issue or problem this excerpt deals with?

b. With regard to this issue or problem, does the excerpt: describe it? tell why it is important? offer a solution?

c. Does the excerpt frame the issue or problem in real-world terms or abstract terms? Or does it only imply the issue or problem?

C. Prescription for revising

Write your prescription for revising to treat the symptoms of *medicus incomprehensibilis*. List the things you would recommend to help improve reading ease and clarity.

D. Revision

Revise the excerpt to improve reading ease and clarity.

1. Looking at *WSEG* scores

Compute the *WSEG* score for your revision. Fill in Table 7-6 to show how your revision compares with the original.

Table 7-6. **Comparing *WSEG* scores**

WSEG		Original	Revised	Change
W	Number of words	180		
S	Average sentence length	30.0		
E	Flesch Reading Ease score	0.0		
G	Flesch-Kincaid Grade Level	23.3		

2. Looking at grammar

Answer the following questions about your revision:

a. Does each sentence put the subject and verb close together within the first 7 or 8 words? If not, tell why it seemed best to do otherwise.

b. Does each sentence use active voice? If not, tell why it seemed best to do otherwise.

c. Does each sentence use a concrete subject? If not, tell why it seemed best to use an abstract subject.

3. Prefer the short word

a. Underline each <u>long word</u>. Count the number of long words and compute long words as a percent of total words. ___ long words / ___ total
words = ___ %. Compare your answer with the percent of long words in
the original. (See §B.4.b.)

b. Double underline any <u>long word</u> you consider a <u>proper name</u> or <u>essential
scientific term</u>.

Notes

1. University of Rochester Medical Center, "Health Encyclopedia: What Are Red Blood Cells?,"
https://www.urmc.rochester.edu/encyclopedia/content.aspx?ContentTypeID=160&Conte
ntID=34 (accessed January 3, 2018).
2. Suetonia Palmer, et al., "Comparison of Clinical Outcomes and Adverse Events Associated
with Glucose-Lowering Drugs in Patients with Type 2 Diabetes: A Meta-analysis," *JAMA*
316, no. 3 (2016): 321–322.
3. Ibid, 314.
4. Diabetes.co.uk, "Guide to HbA1c," https://www.diabetes.co.uk/what-is-hba1c.html
(accessed January 3, 2018).

Glucose Lowering Drugs in Patients with Type 2 Diabetes

Use "active" verbs mainly, not "passive" ones. Using the active is shorter and clearer; using the passive can be longer and sometimes confusing. Try to write 90% in the active. The other 10%—yes, you will find the passive more suitable. —Plain English Campaign (UK), *How to Write Medical Information in Plain English*[1]

A. The excerpt

This case study looks at an excerpt from an article published in *JAMA: The Journal of the American Medical Association*. Read the excerpt out loud:

> <u>Drugs</u> as monotherapy <u>were {associated}</u> with large proportional reductions in HbA$_{1C}$ levels compared with placebo, while metformin was associated with moderately lower HbA$_{1C}$ levels compared with other drugs including sulfonylureas, thiazolidinediones, and DPP-4 inhibitors. Basal <u>insulin and sulfonylureas</u> <u>were {associated}</u> with greatest odds of hypoglycemia, with an absolute risk difference of 10% compared with metformin. <u>Metformin</u> <u>was {associated}</u> with small reductions in body weight relative to sulfonylurea or thiazolidinedione treatment. Considering these results, with metformin showing favorable associations with HbA$_{1C}$ levels compared with sulfonylureas, thiazolidinediones, and DPP-4 inhibitors, and without adverse signals for hypoglycemia or weight gain, <u>metformin</u> <u>might be {considered}</u> a reasonable first-line agent for type 2 diabetes, consistent with the American Diabetes Association recommendations. However, the <u>recommendations</u> also <u>suggested</u> a patient-centered approach—considering efficacy, weight gain, hypoglycemia, and comorbidities—when selecting treatment. Therefore, based on this review, <u>clinicians and patients</u> <u>may prefer</u> to avoid sulfonylureas or basal insulin for patients who wish to minimize hypoglycemia, choose GLP-1 receptor agonists when weight management is a priority, or consider SGLT-2 inhibitors based on their favorable combined safety and efficacy profile. (*WSEG = 180/30.0/0.0/23.3*)

Notes:

1. Metformin, insulins, sulfonylureas, thiazolidinediones, DPP-4 inhibitors, SGLT-2 inhibitors, and GLP-1 receptor agonists are glucose-lowering drug classes approved for type 2 diabetes.

2. HbA_{1C} stands for *hemoglobin A_{1c}* or *glycated hemoglobin*. A hemoglobin molecule glycates when it binds with a glucose molecule. How many glucose molecules bind with a hemoglobin molecule depends on the total glucose in the bloodstream at the time. Since a human red blood cell lives for 8–12 weeks, checking a person's HbA_{1c} level also shows their average blood glucose level over the past 8–12 weeks.

B. Analyzing the excerpt

1. Initial thoughts

What are some of your initial thoughts on this excerpt?

- *Some sentences seem long and cover several ideas.*
- *The paragraph seems long.*
- *The excerpt uses many technical terms that relate to diabetes, how blood glucose is measured, and medicines used to treat diabetes.*
- *Diabetes is an important topic of interest to many people. Understanding diabetes management could be important for a primary care doctor, specialist, nurse, nutritionist, or fitness instructor, among others. But the excerpt seems too technical for some of these people.*

2. Looking at the WSEG score

a. Is the paragraph longer than 150 words? <u>Yes.</u> If so, do you see a good way to split it into shorter paragraphs?

We could split it into two paragraphs. In one paragraph, we could tell about the different drugs used to treat diabetes. Then, in another paragraph, we could say which drug works best in which situation.

b. How does this excerpt's average sentence length compare with the recommended average of 15 words?

It has an average sentence length of 30.0 words—double the recommended average.

c. Count the number of words in each sentence. Then calculate the total number of words. Write your answers in Table 7-1.

Table 7-1. **Words per sentence**

	Sentence						
	1st	*2nd*	*3rd*	*4th*	*5th*	*6th*	*Total*
Number of words	34	21	15	46	18	46	180

d. For each sentence that uses more than 25 words, do you think it needs to be just one long sentence? Why or why not?
The excerpt has three sentences longer than 25 words. They could all be broken up into shorter sentences.

- *First sentence—We could say, in one sentence, that drugs as monotherapy were associated with large proportional reductions in HbA_{1C} compared with placebo. Then, in another sentence, we could say, metformin was associated with moderately lower HbA_{1C} compared with other drugs, including sulfonylureas, thiazolidinediones, and DPP-4 inhibitors.*
- *Fourth sentence—We could say, in one sentence, that metformin showed favorable associations with HbA_{1C} compared with sulfonylureas, thiazolidinediones, and DPP-4 inhibitors. Then, in another sentence, we could say, metformin showed no adverse signals for hypoglycemia or weight gain. Then, in yet another sentence, we can say, metformin might be considered a reasonable first-line agent for type 2 diabetes, consistent with the American Diabetes Association recommendations.*
- *Sixth sentence—We could say, in one sentence, based on this review, clinicians and patients have a number of drug options depending on treatment goals. Then, in another sentence, we could say, patients who wish to minimize hypoglycemia may prefer to avoid sulfonylureas or basal insulin. Then, in yet another sentence, we could say, when weight management is a priority, they may prefer to choose a GLP-1 receptor agonist. Then, in still another sentence, we could say, because of the inhibitor's combined safety and efficacy profile, they may prefer an SGLT-2 inhibitor.*

e. Does the reading ease score fall between 45 and 70 (the one standard deviation range)? <u>No</u>; or between 33 and 83 (the two standard deviation range)? <u>No</u>

f. Does the grade level fall between 6 and 11 (the one standard deviation range)? <u>No</u>; or between 4 and 13 (the two standard deviation range)? <u>No</u>

3. Looking at grammar

a. For each sentence in the excerpt, underline the <u>subject</u> and double underline the <u>main verb</u>. If the main verb includes a past participle, draw braces
around the {past participle}.

b. Fill in Table 7-2, answering the questions for each sentence.

Table 7-2. **Analyze the grammar of each sentence**

Sentence	*Does the main verb contain a form of to be?*	*Is the sentence active, passive or neither?*	*Is the subject abstract or concrete?*	*Are the subject and verb close together in the first 7–8 words?*
1st	yes	passive	concrete	yes
2nd	yes	passive	concrete	yes
3rd	yes	passive	concrete	yes
4th	yes	passive	concrete	no
5th	no	active	abstract	yes
6th	no	active	concrete	no

c. For each abstract subject, explain, in your own words, why it is abstract.
   "Recommendations" are abstract, since they represent ideas.

d. What words or ideas are written in the plural?
   Drugs, reductions, levels, sulfonylureas, thiazolidinediones, inhibitors, odds, reductions, results, associations, signals, recommendations, comorbidities, clinicians, patients, agonists

e. What words or ideas need to be plural?
   Drugs, levels, odds, results, recommendations

f. Fill in Table 7-3 to show your thinking about any phrase that shows possession or connection using *of* or a word ending other than '*s*.

Table 7-3. **Revising phrases that show possession or connection using *of* or a word ending**

List the phrase, underlining <u>*of*</u> *or the* <u>*word* ending</u>	*Is the possession or connection real world or abstract?*	*How might you replace of or the word ending?*
large proportion<u>al</u> reductions	*abstract*	*reduces level more than*
bas<u>al</u> insulin (level)	*abstract*	*(no change—common medical term)*

List the phrase, underlining *of* or the *word* ending	Is the possession or connection real world or abstract?	How might you replace *of* or the word ending?
odds of hypoglycemia	*abstract*	*(no change)*
absolute risk difference of 10%	*abstract*	*risk 10% greater than*
American Diabetes Association	*abstract*	*(no change—proper name)*

4. Prefer the short word

a. Here is a fresh copy of the excerpt. Underline each <u>long word</u>.

> Drugs as <u>monotherapy</u> were <u>associated</u> with large <u>proportional</u> <u>reductions</u> in HbA$_{1c}$ levels compared with <u>placebo</u>, while <u>metformin</u> was <u>associated</u> with <u>moderately</u> lower HbA$_{1c}$ levels compared with other drugs including <u>sulfonylureas</u>, <u>thiazolidinediones</u>, and DPP-4 <u>inhibitors</u>. Basal <u>insulin</u> and <u>sulfonylureas</u> were <u>associated</u> with greatest odds of <u>hypoglycemia</u>, with an <u>absolute</u> risk <u>difference</u> of 10% compared with <u>metformin</u>. <u>Metformin</u> was <u>associated</u> with small <u>reductions</u> in body weight <u>relative</u> to <u>sulfonylurea</u> or <u>thiazolidinedione</u> treatment. <u>Considering</u> these results, with <u>metformin</u> showing <u>favorable</u> <u>associations</u> with HbA$_{1c}$ levels compared with <u>sulfonylureas</u>, <u>thiazolidinediones</u>, and DPP-4 <u>inhibitors</u>, and without adverse signals for <u>hypoglycemia</u> or weight gain, <u>metformin</u> might be <u>considered</u> a <u>reasonable</u> first-line agent for type 2 <u>diabetes</u>, <u>consistent</u> with the <u>American</u> <u>Diabetes</u> <u>Association</u> <u>recommendations</u>. <u>However</u>, the <u>recommendations</u> also suggested a <u>patient-centered</u> approach—<u>considering</u> <u>efficacy</u>, weight gain, <u>hypoglycemia</u>, and <u>comorbidities</u>—when selecting treatment. Therefore, based on this review, <u>clinicians</u> and patients may prefer to avoid <u>sulfonylureas</u> or basal <u>insulin</u> for patients who wish to <u>minimize</u> <u>hypoglycemia</u>, choose GLP-1 <u>receptor</u> <u>agonists</u> when weight <u>management</u> is a <u>priority</u>, or <u>consider</u> SGLT-2 <u>inhibitors</u> based on their <u>favorable</u> combined safety and <u>efficacy</u> profile.

b. Count the number of <u>long words</u> and compute long words as a percent of total words.
<u>61</u> long words/180 total words = <u>33.9</u>%.

c. Double underline any <u>long word</u> you consider a <u>proper name</u> or <u>essential scientific term</u>.

d. For each <u>long word</u> you underlined just once (i.e., skip the essential scientific terms), fill in Table 7-4.

Table 7-4. **Finding shorter words**

Long word	Real world or abstract?	Shorter words that mean about the same thing
monotherapy	real world	one therapy, treat using one method, treat using a single drug, using just one drug
associated	abstract?	connected, linked, causes, leads to, related, tends to
proportional	abstract	in proportion, part, relative, equal, more
reductions	abstract?	reduce, less, lessen, lower, low, drop, cut
moderately	abstract	moderate, a little, slightly, so-so, some, a bit
inhibitors	real world	inhibit, prevent, stop, slow, slow down, block
hypoglycemia	real world	low blood glucose, low blood sugar
difference	abstract?	differ, reduce
relative	abstract?	relate, than, compared to
consider/-ing/-ed	abstract	thought of, thinking about, study, see, look at
favorable	abstract	good, okay
association	abstract?	link, connection, cause, pairing, relate, relation, relationship
reasonable	abstract	good, likely, proper, okay
consistent	abstract	same as, agree, complies with, follows
recommendations	abstract	recommend, guidelines, suggest, advise, instructions, advice
however	abstract	but, yet, in spite of, despite
patient-centered	abstract	personal, for the patient, unique, own, distinct, specific, centered on the patient
efficacy	abstract	effective, effect, how well it works, result
comorbidities	real world	other diseases, have two or more diseases, other illness, sickness
clinicians	real world	doctor or nurse
minimize	abstract	avoid, lower chance of, lessen, make less, reduce
management	abstract	manage, maintain, keep
priority	abstract	goal, first, needed, wanted

e. Look at the long words listed in Table 7-4. Do any of them have the same or a similar meaning?
    - *Associated and association*
    - *Reductions and minimize*
    - *Moderately and reasonable*
    - *Consider and recommendations*
    - *Favorable, reasonable and efficacy*

f. Fill in Table 7-5 by listing each long word that is a nominalization and giving the root verb or adjective.

Table 7-5. **Find the root verb or adjective for each nominalization**

Nominalization	Root verb or adjective
reduction	to reduce
inhibitor	to inhibit
difference	to differ
association	to associate
recommendation	to recommend
efficacy	efficacious
management	to manage
priority	prior

g. Does the excerpt use any compound word(s) whose meaning or pronunciation might be clearer if hyphenated or written as an open compound? If so, tell which one(s) and why you think so.

    We might hyphenate "mono-therapy" and "co-morbidities" so people can better see the two parts.

5. Looking at meaning and logic

a. What is the issue or problem this excerpt deals with?

    Which drugs work best to treat type 2 diabetes, and under what circumstances?

b. With regard to this issue or problem, does the excerpt: describe it? tell why it is important? offer a solution?

    It offers a solution.

c. Does the excerpt frame the issue or problem in real-world terms or abstract terms? Or does it only imply the issue or problem?

    Although the issue and its solution relate mostly to the real world, the excerpt uses many abstract-sounding terms.

C. Prescription for revising

Write your prescription for revising to treat the symptoms of *medicus incomprehensibilis*. List the things you would recommend to help improve reading ease and clarity.

- *Introduce and develop one idea in each paragraph*
- *Keep sentence length 15 words average, 25 words maximum*
- *Revise passive into active voice*
- *Revise abstract into concrete*
- *Observe the 1066 principle*
- *Keep the subject and verb close together in the first 7 or 8 words*
- *Avoid using a high percentage of long words*
- *Keep essential scientific terms; minimize other long words*
- *State the problem before you solve it*
- *Start by anchoring your discussion in the real world*

D. Revision

Revise the excerpt to improve reading ease and clarity.

> We found that treating a patient with just one drug tends to reduce their HbA_{1C} level far more than a _placebo_. _Metformin_ reduces a patient's HbA_{1C} level more than any of the other drugs, including a _sulfonylurea_, a _thiazolidinedione_, or a DPP-4 _inhibitor_.
>
> Basal _insulin_ or a _sulfonylurea_ show the greatest odds of causing low blood glucose. They show an _absolute_ risk that is 10% greater than for _metformin_. A patient who was treated with _metformin_ lost a bit more weight than one treated with a _sulfonylurea_ or a _thiazolidinedione_.
>
> Based on these results, _metformin_ seems to be a good first choice for treating type 2 _diabetes_. It shows better HbA_{1C} levels than a _sulfonylurea_, _thiazolidinedione_, or a DPP-4 _inhibitor_. It also does not tend to cause low blood glucose or weight gain.
>
> This is in keeping with the guidelines of the _American Diabetes Association_. They suggest that treatment should center on the patient. It should _consider_ success in treatment, weight gain, low blood glucose, and any other illness a patient may have.
>
> Therefore, it may be best to avoid a _sulfonylurea_ or basal _insulin_ for a patient who wants to avoid having low blood glucose levels. It may be best to choose a GLP-1 _receptor agonist_ if the patient wants to avoid gaining weight. It may also be worth thinking about an SGLT-2 _inhibitor_, since they tend to be safe and work well.

1. Looking at WSEG scores

Compute the WSEG score for your revision. Fill in Table 7-6 to show how your revision compares with the original.

Table 7-6. **Comparing WSEG scores**

WSEG		Original	Revised	Change
W	Number of words	180	234	54
S	Average sentence length	30.0	16.2	–13.8
E	Flesch Reading Ease score	0.0	55.3	55.3
G	Flesch-Kincaid Grade Level	23.3	9.5	–13.8

2. Looking at grammar

Answer the following questions about your revision:

a. Does each sentence put the subject and verb close together within the first 7 or 8 words? If not, tell why it seemed best to do otherwise.
   Yes.

b. Does each sentence use active voice? If not, tell why it seemed best to do otherwise.
   The revision has several sentences not in active voice.
   - *In paragraph 2, the third sentence is passive. We did this because who is being treated is important, but who does the treating is not.*
   - *In paragraph 4, the first sentence is neither active nor passive. This tracks the original.*
   - *In paragraph 5, the first, second, and third sentences are neither active nor passive. This tracks the original.*

c. Does each sentence use a concrete subject? If not, tell why it seemed best to use an abstract subject.
   The revision uses a number of abstract subjects. The second half of the excerpt deals with general conclusions drawn from analyzing study data. Since the conclusions are general, it seems appropriate they are phrased in abstract terms.

3. Prefer the short word

a. Underline each <u>long word</u>. Count the number of long words and compute long words as a percent of total words. <u>26</u> long words/<u>234</u> total words = <u>11.1</u>%. Compare your answer with the percent of long words in the original. (See §B.4.b.)

b. Double underline any <u>long word</u> you consider a <u>proper name</u> or <u>essential scientific term</u>.

4. Additional comments

Why does our revision use 54 more words than the original?

No one revising decision accounts for the increase. Instead, it resulted from many small choices. The original used long sentences that contained several ideas. Our revision uses shorter sentences that are easier to understand.

The original used abstract language. For our revision, we tried to use more concrete-sounding language. We did this by anchoring the discussion in the real world, using concrete terms, writing in the singular, and talking in terms of one doctor treating one patient.

Our revision used fewer long words than the original (11.1% vs. 33.9%). We kept the essential scientific terms, but replaced other long words with shorter words or a short phrase.

Note

1. Plain English Campaign, "How to Write Medical Information in Plain English," under "Use 'active' verbs mainly, not 'passive' ones," http://www.plainenglish.co.uk/files/medicalguide.pdf (accessed February 5, 2018).

CASE STUDY 8

Low Thyroid Function in Old People

In the active voice, the subject does the acting; in the passive voice,
the subject is acted on. In general, authors should use the active voice,
except in instances in which the actor is unknown or the interest
focuses on what is acted on. —The AMA Manual of Style[1]

A. The excerpt

This case study looks at an excerpt from an article published in *The American Journal of Medicine.*[2] Read the excerpt out loud:

> Organ-specific autoantibodies are rather common among old people. Thus, old age is complicated by an increase in autoimmune disease frequency. Hypothyroidism is no exemption, and in a previous population-based study, we have calculated the median age at disease onset to be 67.6 years. Compared with people aged 0 to 30 years, hypothyroidism was diagnosed 14 times more often in those aged 50 to 60 years, and 33 times more frequently in those aged more than 70 years. This overrules by far the risk associated with female gender, the somewhat higher risk associated with genetic predisposition, and a number of environmental factors, such as iodine intake, smoking habits, alcohol abstinence, and previous live births.
>
> Hypothyroidism may present with a variety of symptoms reflecting the hormonal insufficiency in different organs. However, none of these symptoms have high sensitivity or specificity when compared with euthyroid control persons, and previous studies have suggested scarceness of symptoms specific for hypothyroidism in the older population. Furthermore, old people also may have a variety of other diseases, and the coexistence of thyroid disease and other comorbidities challenges which symptoms may represent which disease. *(WSEG = 186/23.2/19.4/16.3)*

B. Analyzing the excerpt

1. Initial thoughts

What are some of your initial thoughts on this excerpt?

2. Looking at the WSEG score

a. How does this excerpt's average sentence length compare with the recommended average of 15 words?

b. Count the number of words in each sentence. Then calculate the total number of words for each paragraph. Write your answers in Table 8-1.

Table 8-1. **Words per sentence**

		Sentence				
	1st	2nd	3rd	4th	5th	Total
Paragraph 1						
Paragraph 2				—	—	
Grand Total						

c. For each sentence that uses more than 25 words, do you think it needs to be just one long sentence? Why or why not?

d. Does the reading ease score fall between 45 and 70 (the one standard deviation range)?___; or between 33 and 83 (the two standard deviation range)?
e. Does the grade level fall between 6 and 11 (the one standard deviation
   range)?___; or between 4 and 13 (the two standard deviation range)? ___

3. Looking at grammar

a. For each sentence in the excerpt, underline the <u>subject</u> and double underline the <u>main verb</u>. If the main verb includes a past participle, then draw
   braces around the {<u>past participle</u>}.
b. Fill in Table 8-2, answering the questions for each sentence.

Table 8-2. **Analyze the grammar of each sentence**

Sentence	*Does the main verb contain a form of to be?*	*Is the sentence active, passive or neither?*	*Is the subject abstract or concrete?*	*Are the subject and verb close together in the first 7–8 words?*
Paragraph 1				
1st				
2nd				
3rd				
4th				
5th				
Paragraph 2				
1st				
2nd				
3rd				

c. For each abstract subject, explain, in your own words, why it is abstract.

d. What words or ideas are written in the plural?

e. What words or ideas need to be plural?

f. Fill in Table 8-3 to show your thinking about any phrase that shows possession or connection using *of* or a word ending other than *'s*.

Table 8-3. **Revising phrases that show possession or connection using *of* or a word ending**

List the phrase, underlining <u>of</u> or the <u>word</u> ending	Is the possession or connection real world or abstract?	How might you replace of or the word ending?

4. Prefer the short word

a. Here is a fresh copy of the excerpt. Underline each long word.

> Organ-specific autoantibodies are rather common among old people. Thus, old age is complicated by an increase in autoimmune disease frequency. Hypothyroidism is no exemption, and in a previous population-based study, we have calculated the median age at disease onset to be 67.6 years. Compared with people aged 0 to 30 years, hypothyroidism was diagnosed 14 times more often in those aged 50 to 60 years, and 33 times more frequently in those aged more than 70 years. This overrules by far the risk associated with female gender, the somewhat higher risk associated with genetic predisposition, and a number of environmental factors, such as iodine intake, smoking habits, alcohol abstinence, and previous live births.
>
> Hypothyroidism may present with a variety of symptoms reflecting the hormonal insufficiency in different organs. However, none of these symptoms have high sensitivity or specificity when compared with euthyroid control persons, and previous studies have suggested scarceness of symptoms specific for hypothyroidism in the older population. Furthermore, old people also may have a variety of other diseases, and the coexistence of thyroid disease and other comorbidities challenges which symptoms may represent which disease.

b. Count the number of <u>long words</u> and compute long words as a percent of total words.
   ___ long words/186 total words = ___ %.

c. Double underline any <u>long word</u> you consider a <u>proper name</u> or <u>essential scientific term</u>.

d. For each <u>long word</u> you underlined just once (i.e., skip the essential scientific terms), fill in Table 8-4.

Table 8-4. **Finding shorter words**

Long word	Real world or abstract?	Shorter words that mean about the same thing

Long word	Real world or abstract?	Shorter words that mean about the same thing

e. Look at the long words listed in Table 8-4. Do any of them have the same or a similar meaning?

f. Fill in Table 8-5 by listing each long word that is a nominalization and giving the root verb or adjective.

Table 8-5. **Find the root verb or adjective for each nominalization**

Nominalization	Root verb or adjective

g. Does the excerpt use any compound word(s) whose meaning or pronunciation might be clearer if hyphenated or written as an open compound? If so, tell which one(s) and why you think so.

5. Looking at meaning and logic

a. What is the issue or problem this excerpt deals with?

b. With regard to this issue or problem, does the excerpt: describe it? tell why it is important? offer a solution?

c. Does the excerpt frame the issue or problem in real-world terms or abstract terms? Or does it only imply the issue or problem?

C. Prescription for revising

Write your prescription for revising to treat the symptoms of *medicus incomprehensibilis*. List the things you would recommend to help improve reading ease and clarity.

D. Revision

Revise the excerpt to improve reading ease and clarity.

1. Looking at *WSEG* scores

Compute the *WSEG* score for your revision. Fill in Table 8-6 to show how your revision compares with the original.

Table 8-6. **Comparing *WSEG* scores**

WSEG		Original	Revised	Change
W	Number of words	186		
S	Average sentence length	23.2		
E	Flesch Reading Ease score	19.4		
G	Flesch-Kincaid Grade Level	16.3		

2. Looking at grammar

Answer the following questions about your revision:

a. Does each sentence put the subject and verb close together within the first 7 or 8 words? If not, tell why it seemed best to do otherwise.

b. Does each sentence use active voice? If not, tell why it seemed best to do otherwise.

c. Does each sentence use a concrete subject? If not, tell why it seemed best to use an abstract subject.

3. Prefer the short word

a. Underline each <u>long word</u>. Count the number of long words and compute long words as a percent of total words. ___ long words / ___ total words = ___ %. Compare your answer with the percent of long words in the original. (See §B.4.b.)

b. Double underline any <u>long word</u> you consider a <u>proper name</u> or <u>essential scientific term</u>.

Notes

1. Cheryl Iverson et al., *The AMA Manual of Style: A Guide for Authors and Editors*, 10th ed. (New York: Oxford University Press, 2007), sec. 7.3.1.
2. Allan Carlé et al., "Hypothyroid Symptoms Fail to Predict Thyroid Insufficiency in Old People: A Population-Based Case-Controlled Study," *Am J Med* 129, no. 10 (October 2016): 1083.

Low Thyroid Function in Old People

No one should ever have to read a sentence twice because of the way it's put together. —Wilson Follett[1]

A. The excerpt

This case study looks at an excerpt from an article published in *The American Journal of Medicine*. Read the excerpt out loud:

> Organ-specific <u>autoantibodies</u> <u>are</u> rather common among old people. Thus, old <u>age</u> <u>is</u> {complicated} by an increase in autoimmune disease frequency. <u>Hypothyroidism</u> <u>is</u> no exemption, and in a previous population-based study, we have calculated the median age at disease onset to be 67.6 years. Compared with people aged 0 to 30 years, <u>hypothyroidism</u> <u>was</u> {diagnosed} 14 times more often in those aged 50 to 60 years, and 33 times more frequently in those aged more than 70 years. <u>This</u> <u>overrules</u> by far the risk associated with female gender, the somewhat higher risk associated with genetic predisposition, and a number of environmental factors, such as iodine intake, smoking habits, alcohol abstinence, and previous live births.
>
> <u>Hypothyroidism</u> <u>may present</u> with a variety of symptoms reflecting the hormonal insufficiency in different organs. However, <u>none</u> of these symptoms <u>have</u> high sensitivity or specificity when compared with euthyroid control persons, and previous studies have suggested scarceness of symptoms specific for hypothyroidism in the older population. Furthermore, old <u>people</u> also <u>may have</u> a variety of other diseases, and the coexistence of thyroid disease and other comorbidities challenges which symptoms may represent which disease. *(WSEG = 186/23.2/19.4/16.3)*

B. Analyzing the excerpt

1. Initial thoughts

What are some of your initial thoughts on this excerpt?

- *It uses many compound words and other long words.*
- *It uses elegant variation:*
  - *frequency, often, frequently, may*
  - *old people, old age, aged more than 70 years, older population*
  - *other diseases, comorbidities*
- *The fifth sentence, related to environmental risk factors, seems confusing.*

2. Looking at the WSEG score

a. How does this excerpt's average sentence length compare with the recommended average of 15 words?

   It has an average sentence length of 23.3 words—more than 1.5 times the recommended average.

b. Count the number of words in each sentence. Then calculate the total number of words for each paragraph. Write your answers in Table 8-1.

Table 8-1. **Words per sentence**

		Sentence				
	1st	2nd	3rd	4th	5th	Total
Paragraph 1	8	12	23	34	36	113
Paragraph 2	15	31	27	—	—	73
Grand Total						186

c. For each sentence that uses more than 25 words, do you think it needs to be just one long sentence? Why or why not?

   This excerpt has four sentences longer than 25 words. They could all be broken up into shorter sentences.

   Paragraph 1:
   - *Fourth sentence—In one sentence, we could compare people age 0–30 to those age 50–60. Then, in another sentence, we could compare people age 0–30 to those age 70+.*
   - *Fifth sentence—In one sentence, we could say the risk of low thyroid associated with age is overruled by other risk factors. Then, in another sentence, we could list the factors.*

Paragraph 2:

- *Second sentence—We could say, in one sentence, that none of the symptoms have high sensitivity or specificity compared with a control. Then, in another sentence, we could say what previous studies have suggested.*
- *Third sentence—We could say, in one sentence, that old people may have a variety of diseases. Then, in another sentence, we could say that having thyroid disease together with another disease makes it hard to tell which symptom goes with which disease.*

d. Does the reading ease score fall between 45 and 70 (the one standard deviation range)? *No*; or between 33 and 83 (the two standard deviation range)? *No*

e. Does the grade level fall between 6 and 11 (the one standard deviation range)? *No*; or between 4 and 13 (the two standard deviation range)? *No*

3. Looking at grammar

a. For each sentence in the excerpt, underline the <u>subject</u> and double underline the <u>main verb</u>. If the main verb includes a past participle, then draw braces around the {<u>past participle</u>}.

b. Fill in Table 8-2, answering the questions for each sentence.

Table 8-2. **Analyze the grammar of each sentence**

Sentence	*Does the main verb contain a form of to be?*	*Is the sentence active, passive or neither?*	*Is the subject abstract or concrete?*	*Are the subject and verb close together in the first 7–8 words?*
Paragraph 1				
1st	*yes*	*neither*	*concrete*	*yes*
2nd	*yes*	*passive*	*abstract*	*yes*
3rd	*yes*	*neither*	*abstract*	*yes*
4th	*yes*	*passive*	*abstract*	*no*
5th	*no*	*active*	*abstract*	*yes*
Paragraph 2				
1st	*no*	*active*	*abstract*	*yes*
2nd	*no*	*active*	*abstract*	*yes*
3rd	*no*	*active*	*concrete*	*yes*

c. For each abstract subject, explain, in your own words, why it is abstract.
    - *"Age" is abstract because it involves a measurement.*
    - *"Hypothyroidism" is abstract because it is a diagnosis. (Here, the excerpt generalizes about a class of illness. It does not describe a specific patient's illness.)*
    - *"This" (i.e., hypothyroidism being diagnosed more often in certain age ranges) is abstract because it is a generalization about the diagnostic process.*
    - *"None (of these symptoms)" is abstract since it refers to general symptoms, not those specific to hypothyroidism.*

d. What words or ideas are written in the plural?
    Autoantibodies, people, years, times, factors, habits, births, symptoms, organs, persons, studies, diseases, comorbidities, challenges

e. What words or ideas need to be plural?
    People, years, times, factors, births, symptoms, organs, studies, diseases

f. Fill in Table 8-3 to show your thinking about any phrase that shows possession or connection using *of* or a word ending other than *'s*.

Table 8-3. **Revising phrases that show possession or connection using *of* or a word ending**

List the phrase, underlining *of* or the <u>word</u> ending	Is the possession or connection real world or abstract?	How might you replace *of* or the word ending?
geneti<u>c</u> predisposition	*abstract*	*having genes that pre-dispose*
number *of* environment<u>al</u> factors	*abstract*	*many environment<u>al</u> factors*
variety *of* symptoms	*abstract*	*many different symptoms*
none *of* these symptoms	*abstract*	*these symptoms do not*
scarcen<u>ess</u> *of* symptoms	*abstract*	*few symptoms*
variety *of* other diseases	*abstract*	*many other diseases*
coexistence *of* thyroid disease and other comorbidities	*abstract*	*having both thyroid and another disease*

4. Prefer the short word

a. Here is a fresh copy of the excerpt. Underline each long word.

> <u>Organ-specific</u> <u>autoantibodies</u> are rather common among old people. Thus, old age is <u>complicated</u> by an increase in <u>autoimmune</u> disease <u>frequency</u>. <u>Hypothyroidism</u> is no <u>exemption</u>, and in a <u>previous</u> <u>population-based</u> study, we have <u>calculated</u> the <u>median</u> age at disease onset to be 67.6 years. Compared with people aged 0 to 30 years, <u>hypothyroidism</u> was <u>diagnosed</u> 14 times more often in those aged 50 to 60 years, and 33 times more <u>frequently</u> in those aged more than 70 years. This <u>overrules</u> by far the risk <u>associated</u> with female gender, the somewhat higher risk <u>associated</u> with <u>genetic</u> <u>predisposition</u>, and a number of <u>environmental</u> factors, such as <u>iodine</u> intake, smoking habits, <u>alcohol</u> <u>abstinence</u>, and <u>previous</u> live births.
>
> <u>Hypothyroidism</u> may present with a <u>variety</u> of symptoms reflecting the <u>hormonal</u> <u>insufficiency</u> in <u>different</u> organs. <u>However</u>, none of these symptoms have high <u>sensitivity</u> or <u>specificity</u> when compared with <u>euthyroid</u> control persons, and <u>previous</u> studies have suggested scarceness of symptoms <u>specific</u> for <u>hypothyroidism</u> in the older <u>population</u>. <u>Furthermore</u>, old people also may have a <u>variety</u> of other diseases, and the <u>coexistence</u> of thyroid disease and other <u>comorbidities</u> challenges which symptoms may <u>represent</u> which disease.

b. Count the number of <u>long words</u> and compute long words as a percent of total words.
<u>42</u> long words/186 total words = <u>22.6</u>%.

c. Double underline any <u>long word</u> you consider a <u>proper</u> <u>name</u> or <u>essential</u> <u>scientific</u> <u>term</u>.

d. For each <u>long word</u> you underlined just once (i.e., skip the essential scientific terms), fill in Table 8-4.

Table 8-4. **Finding shorter words**

Long word	Real world or abstract?	Shorter words that mean about the same thing
organ-specific	real world	specific to an organ, a certain organ
complicated (by)	abstract	made harder, difficult, complex, another problem
frequency/ frequently	abstract	frequent, often, how often, more often, number of, occurs

Long word	Real world or abstract?	Shorter words that mean about the same thing
hypothyroidism	real world	low thyroid function, under-active thyroid, low thyroid
exemption	abstract	exempt, without, different, except
previous	abstract	past, other, before
population-based	abstract	large-scale study, based on a number of people
calculated	abstract	figured, computed, found
diagnosed	abstract	found, spotted, analyzed
overrules	abstract	outweighs, offsets, eclipses
associated	abstract	linked to, related, connected, from, of
genetic	real world	gene
predisposition	abstract	pre-dispose, susceptible, vulnerable, at risk, at higher risk, tendency, tend to
environmental (factors)	real world	environment, nature, natural, not genetic
abstinence	real world	abstain, do not, avoid, restrict, none, no drinking
variety	abstract	many, different, a number, array
hormonal	real world	hormone
insufficiency	real world?	insufficient, not enough, lacking, low
different	abstract	other
however	abstract	but, yet, in spite of, despite
sensitivity	abstract	sensitive, correct
specificity	abstract	specify, specific, accurate
euthyroid	real world	normal thyroid, good thyroid function
specific	abstract	unique, only, exact, just for
population	real world	group, people
furthermore	abstract	also, likewise, as well, and, too, beyond
coexistence	abstract?	together, both happen at the same time, lives at the same time
comorbidities	real world	other diseases, have two or more diseases, other illness (at the same time)
represent	abstract	belong to, speak for, show, stand for, same

e.   Look at the long words listed in Table 8-4. Do any of them have the same or
a similar meaning?
- *Frequency and frequently*
- *Calculated and diagnosed*
- *Associated and coexistence*
- *Genetic and predisposition*
- *Variety and different*
- *Coexistence and comorbidities*

f.   Fill in Table 8-5 by listing each long word that is a nominalization and
giving the root verb or adjective.

Table 8-5. **Find the root verb or adjective for each nominalization**

Nominalization	Root verb or adjective
frequency	frequent
exemption	to exempt, exempt
predisposition	to (pre-) dispose
abstinence	to abstain
variety	to vary
insufficiency	to (not) suffice
sensitivity	to sense, sensitive
specificity	to specify, specific
population	to populate
coexistence	to (co-) exist
comorbidities	(co-) morbid

g.   Does the excerpt use any compound word(s) whose meaning or pronunciation might be clearer if hyphenated or written as an open compound? If so,
tell which one(s) and why you think so.
*Hypo-thyroidism, pre-disposition, co-existence, co-morbidities, auto-antibodies
and auto-immune would be clearer if written as hyphenated compounds. The
hyphenated forms better reflect pronunciation and meaning.*

5. Looking at meaning and logic

a. What is the issue or problem this excerpt deals with?
    Hypo-thyroidism is an organ-specific auto-immune disease common in old people.
    It can be difficult to diagnose.

b. With regard to this issue or problem, does the excerpt: describe it? tell why
    it is important? offer a solution?
    It describes the problem of hypo-thyroidism in old people.

c. Does the excerpt frame the issue or problem in real-world terms or abstract
    terms? Or does it only imply the issue or problem?
    The excerpt frames the problem of hypo-thyroidism in abstract terms. It
    generalizes about a disease, in a population, over an indefinite time (rather than
    talking about one patient's low thyroid function at a specific time).

C. Prescription for revising

Write your prescription for revising to treat the symptoms of *medicus*
incomprehensibilis. List the things you would recommend to help improve
reading ease and clarity.

- *Keep sentence length 15 words average, 25 words maximum*
- *Don't be afraid to start a sentence with and or but*
- *Omit the needless of*
- *Keep essential scientific terms; minimize other long words*
- *Observe the 1066 principle*
- *Use terms consistently; avoid elegant variation*
- *Write a compound word to promote reading ease and pronunciation*
- *Convert nominalization into a verb in active voice*

D. Revision

Revise the excerpt to improve reading ease and clarity.

> *It is common for an old person to have an <u>auto-antibody</u> that affects just one*
> *organ. Thus, an old person is more likely to have an <u>auto-immune</u> disease.*
> *Low thyroid function is no <u>exception</u>.*
>
> *   In a past large-scale study, we found the <u>median</u> age at disease onset was*
> *67.6 years. Compared with people ages 0 to 30, low thyroid function was*
> *found 14 times more often in those ages 50 to 60. It was found 33 times*
> *more often in those over 70.*

This *overrules* by far other risk factors. These are: female gender, having genes that *pre-dispose*, and *environment* (e.g., *iodine* intake, smoking or drinking habits, and number of live births).

Low thyroid function may present with symptoms that reflect low hormone levels in *different* organs. But none of these symptoms are highly *sensitive* or *specific* when compared to a person with a normal thyroid. Past studies of old people have shown a lack of symptoms specific for low thyroid function.

Old people also may have other diseases. Having both thyroid and some other disease makes it hard to tell which symptom goes with which disease.

1. Looking at WSEG scores

Compute the WSEG score for your revision. Fill in Table 8-6 to show how your revision compares with the original.

Table 8-6. **Comparing WSEG scores**

WSEG		*Original*	*Revised*	*Change*
W	Number of words	186	188	2
S	Average sentence length	23.2	14.4	−8.8
E	Flesch Reading Ease score	19.4	62.1	42.7
G	Flesch-Kincaid Grade Level	16.3	8.1	−8.2

2. Looking at grammar

Answer the following questions about your revision:

a. Does each sentence put the subject and verb close together within the first 7 or 8 words? If not, tell why it seemed best to do otherwise.
No. In paragraph 2, second sentence, we started with the dependent clause, "compared to people 0 to 30 years old," to set up good narrative flow for what follows.

b. Does each sentence use active voice? If not, tell why it seemed best to do otherwise.
No. In paragraph 2, the second and third sentences are in passive voice. The diagnosis of low thyroid function is important, but who makes the diagnosis is not.

c. Does each sentence use a concrete subject? If not, tell why it seemed best to use an abstract subject.
    No. This excerpt generalizes about old people and low thyroid function. Because of the many generalizations, it seemed natural to use abstract subjects.

3. Prefer the short word

a. Underline each <u>long word</u>. Count the number of long words and compute long words as a percent of total words. <u>*11*</u> long words/<u>*188*</u> total words = <u>*5.9*</u>%. Compare your answer with the percent of long words in the original. (See §B.4.b.)
b. Double underline any <u>long word</u> you consider a <u>proper name</u> or <u>essential scientific term</u>.

Note

1. Quoted in Hamilton College, "Writing Tips," https://www.hamilton.edu/tip (accessed October 16, 2016).

Murder Liability for Prescribing Opioids

Communicating clearly is its own reward and saves time and money.
It also improves reader response to messages. Using plain language
avoids creating barriers that set us apart from the people with whom
we are communicating. —National Institutes of Health (USA)[1]

A. The excerpt

This case study looks at an excerpt from an article published in *Mayo Clinic Proceedings.*[2] Read the excerpt out loud:

> As overdoses involving prescription opioids rise, a small but increasing number of physicians face criminal charges for opioid prescribing under state homicide or controlled substance laws or the federal Controlled Substances Act (CSA). Physicians traditionally confront civil medical malpractice suits, restrictions on hospital privileges, and medical board discipline related to patient injuries attributed to their care, including negligent prescribing. But more recently, extreme cases like Dr. Tseng's raise the question: when do physician opioid prescribing behaviors become criminal?
>
> For a prescriber to be criminally (as opposed to civilly) charged, he or she must exhibit a blameworthy, or culpable, state of mind. Murder charges under state homicide laws can follow when a physician engages in risky opioid prescribing that is likely to result in an adverse consequence, such as death, *purposefully* or with a *subjective understanding* of the risks (Table). Lesser involuntary manslaughter (sometimes termed "criminal negligence") charges require *reckless* prescribing, where the prescribers should have been aware of the risks but evidence suggests they subjectively did not appreciate them (Table). Under CSA and many comparable state controlled substance laws, it is a crime to prescribe controlled substances, such as opioids, for reasons other than a legitimate medical purpose and in the usual course of professional practice (Table). (*WSEG = 207/29.5/16.6/18.2*)

B. Analyzing the excerpt

1. Initial thoughts

What are some of your initial thoughts on this excerpt?

2. Looking at the WSEG score

a. How does this excerpt's average sentence length compare with the recommended average of 15 words?

b. Count the number of words in each sentence. Then calculate the total number of words for each paragraph. Write your answers in Table 9-1.

Table 9-1. **Words per sentence**

	Sentence				
	1st	*2nd*	*3rd*	*4th*	*Total*
Paragraph 1					
Paragraph 2					
Grand Total					

c. Is any paragraph longer than 150 words? ____ If so, do you see a good way to split it into shorter paragraphs?

d. For each sentence that uses more than 25 words, do you think it needs to be just one long sentence? Why or why not?

e. Does the reading ease score fall between 45 and 70 (the one standard deviation range)?___; or between 33 and 83 (the two standard deviation range)? ___

f. Does the grade level fall between 6 and 11 (the one standard deviation range)?___; or between 4 and 13 (the two standard deviation range)? ___

3. Looking at grammar

a. For each sentence in the excerpt, underline the <u>subject</u> and double underline the <u>main verb</u>. If the main verb includes a past participle, then draw braces around the {<u>past participle</u>}.

b. Fill in Table 9-2, answering the questions for each sentence.

Table 9-2. **Analyze the grammar of each sentence**

Sentence	*Does the main verb contain a form of to be?*	*Is the sentence active, passive or neither?*	*Is the subject abstract or concrete?*	*Are the subject and verb close together in the first 7–8 words?*
Paragraph 1				
1st				
2nd				
3rd				

Sentence	Does the main verb contain a form of to be?	Is the sentence active, passive or neither?	Is the subject abstract or concrete?	Are the subject and verb close together in the first 7–8 words?
Paragraph 2				
1st				
2nd				
3rd				
4th				

c. For each abstract subject, explain, in your own words, why it is abstract.

d. What words or ideas are written in the plural?

e. What words or ideas need to be plural?

f. Fill in Table 9-3 to show your thinking about any phrase that shows possession or connection using *of* or a word ending other than *'s*.

Table 9-3. **Revising phrases that show possession or connection using *of* or a word ending**

List the phrase, underlining *of* or the *word ending*	Is the possession or connection real world or abstract?	How might you replace *of* or the word ending?

4. Prefer the short word

a. Here is a fresh copy of the excerpt. Underline each <u>long word</u>.

> As overdoses involving prescription opioids rise, a small but increasing number of physicians face criminal charges for opioid prescribing under state homicide or controlled substance laws or the federal Controlled Substances Act (CSA). Physicians traditionally confront civil medical malpractice suits, restrictions on hospital privileges, and medical board discipline related to patient injuries attributed to their care, including negligent prescribing. But more recently, extreme cases like Dr. Tseng's raise the question: when do physician opioid prescribing behaviors become criminal?
>
> For a prescriber to be criminally (as opposed to civilly) charged, he or she must exhibit a blameworthy, or culpable, state of mind. Murder charges under state homicide laws can follow when a physician engages in risky opioid prescribing that is likely to result in an adverse consequence, such as death, *purposefully* or with a *subjective understanding* of the risks (Table). Lesser involuntary manslaughter (sometimes termed "criminal negligence") charges require *reckless* prescribing, where the prescribers should have been aware of the risks but evidence suggests they subjectively did not appreciate them (Table). Under CSA and many comparable state controlled substance laws, it is a crime to prescribe controlled substances, such as opioids, for reasons other than a legitimate medical purpose and in the usual course of professional practice (Table).

b. Count the number of <u>long words</u> and compute long words as a percent of total words.
   ___ long words/207 total words = ___ %.
c. Double underline any <u>long word</u> you consider a <u>proper</u> <u>name</u> or <u>essential scientific</u> <u>term</u>.
d. For each <u>long word</u> you underlined just once (i.e., skip the essential scientific terms), fill in Table 9-4.

Table 9-4. **Finding shorter words**

Long word	Real world or abstract?	Shorter words that mean about the same thing

Long word	Real world or abstract?	Shorter words that mean about the same thing

e. Look at the long words listed in Table 9-4. Do any of them have the same or a similar meaning?

f. Fill in Table 9-5 by listing each long word that is a nominalization and giving the root verb or adjective.

Table 9-5. **Find the root verb or adjective for each nominalization**

Nominalization	Root verb or adjective

g. Does the excerpt use any compound word(s) whose meaning or pronunciation might be clearer if hyphenated or written as an open compound? If so, tell which one(s) and why you think so.

5. Looking at meaning and logic

a. What is the issue or problem this excerpt deals with?

b. With regard to this issue or problem, does the excerpt: describe it? tell why it is important? offer a solution?

c. Does the excerpt frame the issue or problem in real-world terms or abstract terms? Or does it only imply the issue or problem?

C. Prescription for revising

Write your prescription for revising to treat the symptoms of *medicus incomprehensibilis*. List the things you would recommend to help improve reading ease and clarity.

D. Revision

Revise the excerpt to improve reading ease and clarity.

1. Looking at *WSEG* scores

Compute the *WSEG* score for your revision. Fill in Table 9-6 to show how your revision compares with the original.

Table 9-6. **Comparing *WSEG* scores**

WSEG		*Original*	*Revised*	*Change*
W	Number of words	207		
S	Average sentence length	29.5		
E	Flesch Reading Ease score	16.6		
G	Flesch-Kincaid Grade Level	18.2		

2. Looking at grammar

Answer the following questions about your revision:

a. Does each sentence put the subject and verb close together within the first 7 or 8 words? If not, tell why it seemed best to do otherwise.

b. Does each sentence use active voice? If not, tell why it seemed best to do otherwise.

c. Does each sentence use a concrete subject? If not, tell why it seemed best to use an abstract subject.

3. Prefer the short word

a. Underline each <u>long word</u>. Count the number of <u>long words</u> and compute long words as a percent of total words. ____ long words / ____ total words = ____ %. Compare your answer with the percent of long words in the original. (See §B.4.b.)

b. Double underline any <u>long word</u> you consider a <u>proper name</u> or <u>essential scientific term</u>.

Notes

1. National Institute of Health, "Plain Language at NIH," https://www.nih.gov/institutes-nih/nih-office-director/office-communications-public-liaison/clear-communication/plain-language (accessed February 5, 2018).
2. Tony Yang and Rebecca Haffajee, "Murder Liability for Prescribing Opioids: A Way Forward?" *Mayo Clinic Proc* 91, no. 10 (October 2016): 1331, 1333.

Murder Liability for Prescribing Opioids

Refining a text is laborious and time consuming. . . . If you consistently train yourself, little by little, to observe these rules, however, they will become automatic. Realizing that you are doing this spontaneously is satisfying because you know you are saving time and writing better at the same time. —Alistair Reeves, "Time to Make It Shorter: Plain English in Our Context"[1]

A. The excerpt

This case study looks at an excerpt from an article published in *Mayo Clinic Proceedings*. Read the excerpt out loud:

As overdoses involving prescription opioids rise, a small but increasing <u>number</u> of physicians <u>face</u> criminal charges for opioid prescribing under state homicide or controlled substance laws or the federal Controlled Substances Act (CSA). <u>Physicians</u> traditionally <u>confront</u> civil medical malpractice suits, restrictions on hospital privileges, and medical board discipline related to patient injuries attributed to their care, including negligent prescribing. But more recently, extreme <u>cases</u> like Dr. Tseng's <u>raise</u> the question: when do physician opioid prescribing behaviors become criminal?

For a prescriber to be criminally (as opposed to civilly) charged, <u>he or she</u> <u>must exhibit</u> a blameworthy, or culpable, state of mind. Murder <u>charges</u> under state homicide laws <u>can follow</u> when a physician engages in risky opioid prescribing that is likely to result in an adverse consequence, such as death, *purposefully* or with a *subjective understanding* of the risks (Table). Lesser involuntary manslaughter (sometimes termed "criminal negligence") <u>charges</u> <u>require</u> *reckless* prescribing, where the prescribers should have been aware of the risks but evidence suggests they subjectively did not appreciate them (Table). Under CSA and many comparable state controlled substance laws, <u>it is</u> a crime to prescribe controlled substances, such as opioids, for reasons other than a legitimate medical purpose and in the usual course of professional practice (Table). (*WSEG = 207/29.5/16.6/18.2*)

B. Analyzing the excerpt

1. Initial thoughts

What are some of your initial thoughts on this excerpt?
- *The sentences seem long.*
- *This article is about US law, as opposed to medical science. It uses more legal terms than medical terms.*
- *This article might interest anyone prescribing opioids in the United States. Doctors in other countries would probably find it less interesting.*

2. Looking at the WSEG score

a. How does this excerpt's average sentence length compare with the recommended average of 15 words?
   It has an average sentence length of 29.5 words—almost twice the recommended average.
b. Count the number of words in each sentence. Then calculate the total number of words for each paragraph. Write your answers in Table 9-1.

Table 9-1. **Words per sentence**

	Sentence				
	1st	*2nd*	*3rd*	*4th*	*Total*
Paragraph 1	33	26	19	—	78
Paragraph 2	23	38	31	37	129
Grand Total					207

c. Is any paragraph longer than 150 words? <u>No</u>. If so, do you see a good way to split it into shorter paragraphs?
   N/A
d. For each sentence that uses more than 25 words, do you think it needs to be just one long sentence? Why or why not?
   The excerpt has five sentences longer than 25 words. Most can be broken up into shorter sentences.
   Paragraph 1:
   - *First sentence—We could say, in one sentence, that overdoses are on the rise. In another sentence, we could say that the number of doctors being charged has increased. Then, in yet another sentence, we could say the doctors are being changed under state homicide and controlled substance laws or the federal Controlled Substances Act (CSA).*

- *Second sentence—We could say, in one sentence, a doctor may face civil claims. Then, in another sentence, we could say what those claims may be.*

  Paragraph 2:

- *Second sentence—We could say, in one sentence, that murder charges may follow. Then, in another sentence, we could say that, to be charged, the doctor must have acted "purposefully" or with a "subjective understanding" of the risks.*

- *Third sentence—We could say, in one sentence, that involuntary manslaughter involves reckless prescribing. Then, in another sentence, we could define reckless prescribing.*

- *Fourth sentence—Since this sentence is just one idea and quotes the language of the CSA, we would leave it as one sentence (but would try to shorten it if possible).*

e. Does the reading ease score fall between 45 and 70 (the one standard deviation range)? <u>No</u>; or between 33 and 83 (the two standard deviation range)? <u>No</u>

f. Does the grade level fall between 6 and 11 (the one standard deviation range)? <u>No</u>; or between 4 and 13 (the two standard deviation range)? <u>No</u>

3. Looking at grammar

a. For each sentence in the excerpt, underline the <u>subject</u> and double underline the <u>main verb</u>. If the main verb includes a past participle, then draw braces around the {<u>past participle</u>}.

b. Fill in Table 9-2, answering the questions for each sentence.

Table 9-2. **Analyze the grammar of each sentence**

Sentence	Does the main verb contain a form of to be?	Is the sentence active, passive or neither?	Is the subject abstract or concrete?	Are the subject and verb close together in the first 7–8 words?
Paragraph 1				
1st	*no*	*active*	*abstract*	*no*
2nd	*no*	*active*	*concrete*	*yes*
3rd	*no*	*active*	*abstract*	*no*

Sentence	Does the main verb contain a form of to be?	Is the sentence active, passive or neither?	Is the subject abstract or concrete?	Are the subject and verb close together in the first 7–8 words?
Paragraph 2				
1st	*no*	*active*	*concrete*	*no*
2nd	*no*	*active*	*abstract*	*yes*
3rd	*no*	*active*	*abstract*	*no*
4th	*yes*	*neither*	*abstract*	*no*

c. For each abstract subject, explain, in your own words, why it is abstract.
   - *"Number" is a generalization.*
   - *"Cases"—A legal case involves many real-world actions guided by abstract thought and analysis.*
   - *"Charges" are formal accusations (i.e., ideas) that a person has broken the law.*
   - *"It" (prescribing controlled substances without a medical reason) involves both a real-world action and the thought process behind it.*

d. What words or ideas are written in the plural?
   Overdoses, opioids, physicians, charges, laws, Substances, suits, restrictions, privileges, injuries, cases, behaviors, risks, prescribers, reasons

e. What words or ideas need to be plural?
   Overdoses, physicians, charges, laws, Substances, privileges, cases, risks

f. Fill in Table 9-3 to show your thinking about any phrase that shows possession or connection using *of* or a word ending other than *'s.*

Table 9-3. **Revising phrases that show possession or connection using *of* or a word ending**

List the phrase, underlining *of* or the <u>word</u> <u>ending</u>	Is the possession or connection real world or abstract?	How might you replace *of* or the word ending?
number of physicians	*abstract*	*(no change)*
state of mind	*abstract*	*(no change—legal term)*
subjective understanding of the risks	*abstract*	*(no change)*
should have been aware of the risks	*abstract*	*should have known the risks*
usual course of professional practice	*abstract*	*(no change)*

4. Prefer the short word

a. Here is a fresh copy of the excerpt. Underline each <u>long word</u>.

> As <u>overdoses</u> involving <u>prescription</u> <u>opioids</u> rise, a small but increasing number of <u>physicians</u> face <u>criminal</u> charges for <u>opioid</u> prescribing under state <u>homicide</u> or controlled substance laws or the <u>federal</u> Controlled Substances Act (CSA). <u>Physicians</u> <u>traditionally</u> confront civil <u>medical</u> <u>malpractice</u> suits, <u>restrictions</u> on <u>hospital</u> <u>privileges</u>, and <u>medical</u> board <u>discipline</u> related to patient <u>injuries</u> <u>attributed</u> to their care, including <u>negligent</u> prescribing. But more <u>recently</u>, extreme cases like Dr. Tseng's raise the question: when do <u>physician</u> <u>opioid</u> prescribing <u>behaviors</u> become <u>criminal</u>?
>
> For a <u>prescriber</u> to be <u>criminally</u> (as opposed to <u>civilly</u>) charged, he or she must <u>exhibit</u> a <u>blameworthy</u>, or <u>culpable</u>, state of mind. Murder charges under state <u>homicide</u> laws can follow when a <u>physician</u> engages in risky <u>opioid</u> prescribing that is likely to result in an adverse <u>consequence</u>, such as death, *<u>purposefully</u>* or with a *<u>subjective</u>* *<u>understanding</u>* of the risks (Table). Lesser <u>involuntary</u> <u>manslaughter</u> (sometimes termed "<u>criminal</u> <u>negligence</u>") charges require *reckless* prescribing, where the <u>prescribers</u> should have been aware of the risks but <u>evidence</u> suggests they <u>subjectively</u> did not <u>appreciate</u> them (Table). Under CSA and many <u>comparable</u> state controlled substance laws, it is a crime to prescribe controlled substances, such as <u>opioids</u>, for reasons other than a <u>legitimate</u> <u>medical</u> purpose and in the usual course of <u>professional</u> practice (Table).

b. Count the number of <u>long words</u> and compute long words as a percent of total words.
    <u>51</u> long words/207 total words = <u>24.6</u>%.
c. Double underline any <u>long word</u> you consider a <u>proper name</u> or <u>essential scientific term</u>.
d. For each <u>long word</u> you underlined just once (i.e., skip the essential scientific terms), fill in Table 9-4.

Table 9-4. **Finding shorter words**

Long word	Real world or abstract?	Shorter words that mean about the same thing
overdoses	*real world*	*take too much, too high a dose, harmful dose, fatal dose, more than prescribed, more than the doctor orders*

Long word	Real world or abstract?	Shorter words that mean about the same thing
prescription	abstract	prescribe, legal, controlled, ordered by the doctor
physicians	real world	doctor
criminal	abstract	crime, break the law, not legal
federal	abstract	national, US
traditionally	abstract	traditional, usually, often, most of the time, before, in the old days
medical	abstract	healthcare, licensing
restrictions	abstract	restrict, take away, lessen, reduce
hospital	real world	clinic, admitting, admit
privileges	abstract	permission, allowed, license, okay, permit, can, rights
discipline	abstract	restraint, censure, punish, sanction, fine, restrict
injuries	real world	injure, hurt, harm, wounds
attributed	abstract	connect, trace, credit, from, because
negligent	abstract	careless, wrong, wrongful, not legal, mistake
recently	abstract	lately, recent, new, now
behaviors	abstract	action, work, practice
prescriber	real world	doctor, one who prescribes
criminally	abstract	criminal, crime
civilly	abstract	civil, break a rule
exhibit	abstract	show, have
blameworthy	abstract	worthy of blame, at fault, guilty, guilt
culpable	abstract	meriting blame, at fault, guilty, guilt
consequence	abstract	result, ending, effect, end, outcome
purposefully	abstract	on purpose, not by mistake, intend, actively, knowing, knowingly
subjective	abstract	one's own
understanding	abstract	understand, know, knowledge, aware
evidence	abstract	data, proof, fact, finding
subjectively	abstract	personal, actual

Long word	Real world or abstract?	Shorter words that mean about the same thing
appreciate	abstract	respect, acknowledge, take into account, know, know of, understand, accept, like
comparable	abstract	compare, similar, like, other
legitimate	abstract	real, actual, accepted, understood, good faith, legal, lawful, true
professional	abstract	medical, doctor

e. Look at the long words listed in Table 9-4. Do any of them have the same or a similar meaning?
   • *Physicians, prescribers and professional*
   • *Traditionally and legitimate*
   • *Medical and professional*
   • *Blameworthy, culpable, criminally, discipline, criminal and civilly*
   • *Purposefully, subjective and subjectively*
   • *Understanding and appreciate*

f. Fill in Table 9-5 by listing each long word that is a nominalization and giving the root verb or adjective.

Table 9-5. **Find the root verb or adjective for each nominalization**

Nominalization	Root verb or adjective
overdose	to overdose, to dose, over
prescription, prescriber	to prescribe
restriction	to restrict
discipline	to discipline
injuries	to injure
behavior	to behave
understanding	to understand

g. Does the excerpt use any compound word(s) whose meaning or pronunciation might be clearer if hyphenated or written as an open compound? If so, tell which one(s) and why you think so.
   No.

5. Looking at meaning and logic

a. What is the issue or problem this excerpt deals with?
   When do physician opioid prescribing behaviors become criminal?
b. With regard to this issue or problem, does the excerpt: describe it? tell why
   it is important? offer a solution?
   It states the question and answers it.
c. Does the excerpt frame the issue or problem in real-world terms or abstract
   terms? Or does it only imply the issue or problem?
   *It frames the issue in abstract terms. It generalizes about facts, and talks about
   laws (which are, by their nature, abstract).*

C. Prescription for revising

Write your prescription for revising to treat the symptoms of *medicus
incomprehensibilis*. List the things you would recommend to help improve
reading ease and clarity.
- *Keep sentence length 15 words average, 25 words maximum*
- *Introduce and develop one idea in each paragraph*
- *Keep the subject and verb close together in the first 7 or 8 words*
- *Revise abstract into concrete*
- *Write in the singular*
- *Keep essential scientific terms; minimize other long words*
- *Convert nominalization into a verb in active voice*

D. Revision

Revise the excerpt to improve reading ease and clarity.

> *Overdoses involving prescription opioids are rising. A small but growing
> number of doctors face criminal charges for opioid prescribing. These charges
> are brought under state homicide or controlled substance laws, or the fed-
> eral Controlled Substances Act (CSA).*
>
> *It has long been the case that a doctor might face a civil claim if their care
> injures a patient. This could include a malpractice lawsuit, restricted hos-
> pital privileges, or medical board discipline. But lately, cases like Dr. Tseng's
> raise a new question. When does prescribing an opioid become a crime?*
>
> *For a doctor to commit a crime, they must show a blameworthy state of
> mind. A murder charge under a state law can follow if the doctor engages in
> risky opioid prescribing that is likely to lead to the patient's death or some*

other bad result. In order to be guilty of a crime, the doctor must act <u>*pur-</u>
<u>*posefully*</u> or with a <u>*subjective*</u> <u>*understanding*</u> of the risks (Table).

Involuntary manslaughter charges require reckless prescribing. This
means the doctor knew, or should have known, the risk but <u>*evidence*</u> shows
they did not (Table). This is sometimes termed "<u>*criminal*</u> <u>*negligence*</u>."

Under the CSA and many state laws, it is a crime to prescribe a controlled
substance, such as an <u>*opioid*</u>, without a <u>*legitimate*</u> <u>*medical*</u> purpose or outside the usual course of <u>*medical*</u> practice (Table).

1. Looking at WSEG scores

Compute the WSEG score for your revision. Fill in Table 9-6 to show how your
revision compares with the original.

Table 9-6. **Comparing WSEG scores**

WSEG		*Original*	*Revised*	*Change*
W	Number of words	207	220	13
S	Average sentence length	29.5	15.7	–13.8
E	Flesch Reading Ease score	16.6	55.9	39.3
G	Flesch-Kincaid Grade Level	18.2	9.3	–8.9

2. Looking at grammar

Answer the following questions about your revision:

a. Does each sentence put the subject and verb close together within the first
7 or 8 words? If not, tell why it seemed best to do otherwise.
   No.
   Paragraph 3:
   • *First sentence—the subject, "they," and verb, "must show," are close to-
     gether; but the sentence starts with an introductory phrase, which keeps
     them from being in the first 7 or 8 words.*
   • *Second sentence—the subject, "charge," and verb, "can follow," are separated
     by information about the charge.*

- *Third sentence—the subject, "doctors," and verb, "must act," are close to-gether; but the sentence starts with an introductory phrase, which keeps them from being in the first 7 or 8 words.*
  Paragraph 5:
- *First sentence—the subject, "it," and verb, "is," are close together; but the sentence starts with an introductory phrase, which keeps them from being in the first 7 or 8 words.*

b. Does each sentence use active voice? If not, tell why it seemed best to do otherwise.

No. We had a few sentences that do not use active voice.

- *Paragraph 1, first sentence is neither active nor passive. This follows the meaning of the original.*
- *Paragraph 1, third sentence is passive. The laws under which the charges are brought are important, but who brings the charges is not.*
- *Paragraph 2, first sentence is neither active nor passive. "It has long been the case" seemed better than "traditionally."*
- *Paragraph 4, third sentence is passive. What the crime is called is impor-tant, but who does the calling is not.*
- *Paragraph 5, first sentence is neither active nor passive. It describes what constitutes a crime.*

c. Does each sentence use a concrete subject? If not, tell why it seemed best to use an abstract subject.

No. This excerpt talks about an abstract topic, legal analysis. Because of this, our revision used several abstract subjects.

3. Prefer the short word

a. Underline each <u>long word</u>. Count the number of <u>long words</u> and compute long words as a percent of total words. <u>27</u> long words/<u>220</u> total words = <u>12.3</u>%. Compare your answer with the percent of long words in the original. (See §B.4.b.)

b. Double underline any <u>long word</u> you consider a <u>proper name</u> or <u>essential scientific term</u>.

Note

1. Alistair Reeves, "Time to Make It Shorter: Plain English in Our Context," *Medical Writing* 24, no. 1 (2015): 6.; The "rules" mentioned here are from George Orwell's essay, "Politics and the English Language," *Horizon* 13, no. 76 (1964). Specifically, Reeves is referring to rules 2 and 3: "Never use a long word where a short one will do," and "If it is possible to cut out a word, always cut it out."

CASE STUDY 10

Factors Associated with Preventable Re-Admissions

An active voice sentence clearly identifies the action and who is performing that action. The active voice is more to the point and lively. Unfortunately, a lot of writing uses the passive voice, which gives documents a wordy, bureaucratic tone. —Writing in Plain Language, The Royal Children's Hospital of Melbourne (Australia)[1]

A. The excerpt

This case study looks at an excerpt from an article published in *JAMA Internal Medicine*.[2] The article tells about a study of 1,000 general medicine patients re-admitted within 30 days of discharge. Of these re-admissions, 269 were considered *preventable*, and the other 731 *non-preventable*. This excerpt describes factors associated with potentially preventable re-admissions. Read the excerpt out loud:

> Multiple potential underlying factors were noted when we compared preventable and nonpreventable readmissions in the domains of medication safety, care coordination, discharge planning, advance care planning, promotion of self-management, enlisting of help and social supports, diagnostic and therapeutic problems, and monitoring and managing of symptoms after discharge. Of potential underlying factors, those variables with the largest absolute differences in prevalence between preventable and nonpreventable readmissions were the following: inadequate treatment of symptoms other than pain (20.8% [56 of 269] vs 6.4% [47 of 731]), inadequate monitoring for medication adverse effects or nonadherence (14.9% [40 of 269] vs 4.4% [32 of 731]), follow-up appointments not scheduled sufficiently soon after discharge (16.0% [43 of 269] vs 5.7% [42 of 731]), patient lack of awareness of whom to contact after discharge or when to go (or not to go) to the emergency department (18.6% [50 of 269] vs 5.7% [42 of 731]), patient need for additional or different home services than those services included in discharge plans (17.8% [48 of 269] vs 7.8% [57 of 731]), discharge of patients too soon (eg, symptoms such

as inability to eat or dyspnea not completely managed) from the index hospitalization (19.3% [52 of 269] vs 4.0% [29 of 731]), and issues related to the decision to admit the patient made in the emergency department (eg, the patient may not have required an inpatient stay, or useful information from the primary care physician was not available or reviewed) (12.6% [34 of 269] vs 2.6% [19 of 731]) (Table 4). *(WSEG = 252/126.0/0.0/57.5)*

Note: "Table 4," mentioned at the end of the excerpt, lists all of the potential underlying factors that lead to re-admissions, together with their related data. The factors are grouped by domain.

B. Analyzing the excerpt

1. Initial thoughts

What are some of your initial thoughts on this excerpt?

2. Looking at the WSEG score

a. Is the paragraph longer than 150 words? ____ If so, do you see a good way to split it into shorter paragraphs?

b. How does this excerpt's average sentence length compare with the recommended average of 15 words?

c. How many words does each sentence use? First ____, second ____

d. For each sentence that uses more than 25 words, do you think it needs to be just one long sentence? Why or why not?

e. Does the reading ease score fall between 45 and 70 (the one standard deviation range)? ___; or between 33 and 83 (the two standard deviation range)? ___

f. Does the grade level fall between 6 and 11 (the one standard deviation range)? ___; or between 4 and 13 (the two standard deviation range)? ___

3. Looking at grammar

a. For each sentence in the excerpt, underline the <u>subject</u> and double underline the <u>main verb</u>. If the main verb includes a past participle, then draw braces around the {<u>past participle</u>}.

b. Fill in Table 10-1, answering the questions for each sentence.

Table 10-1. **Analyze the grammar of each sentence**

Sentence	*Does the main verb contain a form of to be?*	*Is the sentence active, passive or neither?*	*Is the subject abstract or concrete?*	*Are the subject and verb close together in the first 7–8 words?*
1st				
2nd				

c. For each abstract subject, explain, in your own words, why it is abstract.

d. What words or ideas are written in the plural?

e. What words or ideas need to be plural?

f. Fill in Table 10-2 to show your thinking about any phrase that shows possession or connection using *of* or a word ending other than '*s*.

Table 10-2. **Revising phrases that show possession or connection using** *of* **or a word ending**

List the phrase, underlining <u>of</u> or the <u>word ending</u>	Is the possession or connection real world or abstract?	How might you replace *of* or the word ending?

4. Prefer the short word

a. Here is a fresh copy of the excerpt. Underline each <u>long word</u>.

> Multiple potential underlying factors were noted when we compared preventable and nonpreventable readmissions in the domains of medication safety, care coordination, discharge planning, advance care planning, promotion of self-management, enlisting of help and social supports, diagnostic and therapeutic problems, and monitoring and managing of symptoms after discharge. Of potential underlying factors, those variables with the largest absolute differences in prevalence between preventable and nonpreventable readmissions were the following: inadequate treatment of symptoms other than pain (20.8% [56 of 269] vs 6.4% [47 of 731]), inadequate monitoring for medication adverse effects or nonadherence (14.9% [40 of 269] vs 4.4% [32 of 731]), follow-up appointments not scheduled sufficiently soon after discharge (16.0% [43 of 269] vs 5.7% [42 of 731]), patient lack

of awareness of whom to contact after discharge or when to go (or not to go) to the emergency department (18.6% [50 of 269] vs 5.7% [42 of 731]), patient need for additional or different home services than those services included in discharge plans (17.8% [48 of 269] vs 7.8% [57 of 731]), discharge of patients too soon (eg, symptoms such as inability to eat or dyspnea not completely managed) from the index hospitalization (19.3% [52 of 269] vs 4.0% [29 of 731]), and issues related to the decision to admit the patient made in the emergency department (eg, the patient may not have required an inpatient stay, or useful information from the primary care physician was not available or reviewed) (12.6% [34 of 269] vs 2.6% [19 of 731]) (Table 4).

b. Count the number of <u>long words</u> and compute long words as a percent of total words.

_____ long words/252 total words = ____%.

c. Double underline any <u>long word</u> you consider a <u>proper</u> <u>name</u> or <u>essential</u> <u>scientific</u> <u>term</u>.

d. For each <u>long word</u> you underlined just once (i.e., skip the essential scientific terms), fill in Table 10-3.

Table 10-3. **Finding shorter words**

Long word	Real world or abstract?	Shorter words that mean about the same thing

Long word	Real world or abstract?	Shorter words that mean about the same thing

e. Look at the long words listed in Table 10-3. Do any of them have the same or a similar meaning?

f. Fill in Table 10-4 by listing each long word that is a nominalization and giving the root verb or adjective.

Table 10-4. **Find the root verb or adjective for each nominalization**

Nominalization	Root verb or adjective

g. Does the excerpt use any compound word(s) whose meaning or pronunciation might be clearer if hyphenated or written as an open compound? If so, tell which one(s) and why you think so.

5. Looking at meaning and logic

a. What is the issue or problem this excerpt deals with?

b. With regard to this issue or problem, does the excerpt: describe it? tell why it is important? offer a solution?

c. Does the excerpt frame the issue or problem in real-world terms or abstract terms? Or does it only imply the issue or problem?

C. Prescription for revising

Write your prescription for revising to treat the symptoms of *medicus incomprehensibilis*. List the things you would recommend to help improve reading ease and clarity.

- *Omit the numerical data (which is repeated in Table 4 mentioned in the excerpt)*

D. Revision

Revise the excerpt to improve reading ease and clarity. In your revision, omit the numerical data (which is repeated in Table 4). Consider using tables, bullet points, or numbered lists in your revision.

1. Looking at WSEG scores

Compute the WSEG score for your revision. Fill in Table 10-5 to show how your revision compares with the original.

Table 10-5. **Comparing WSEG scores**

WSEG		Original	Revised	Change
W	Number of words	252		
S	Average sentence length	126.0		
E	Flesch Reading Ease score	0.0		
G	Flesch-Kincaid Grade Level	57.5		

2. Looking at grammar

Answer the following questions about your revision:

a. Does each sentence put the subject and verb close together within the first 7 or 8 words? If not, tell why it seemed best to do otherwise.

b. Does each sentence use active voice? If not, tell why it seemed best to do otherwise.

c. Does each sentence use a concrete subject? If not, tell why it seemed best to use an abstract subject.

3. Prefer the short word

a. Underline each long word. Count the number of long words and compute long words as a percent of total words. ___ long words / ___ total words = ___ %. Compare your answer with the percent of long words in the original. (See §B.4.b.)

b. Double underline any long word you consider a proper name or essential scientific term.

Notes

1. The Royal Children's Hospital of Melbourne, "Writing in Plain Language," under "Favour the active voice," http://www.rch.org.au/uploadedFiles/Main/Content/ethics/Writing%20 Tips.pdf (accessed February 5, 2018).
2. Andrew Auerbach et al., "Preventability and Causes of Readmissions in a National Cohort of General Medicine Patients," *JAMA Internal Medicine* 176, no. 4 (April 2016): 488.

Factors Associated with Preventable Re-Admissions

As a starting point and at every point, design and write the document in a way that best serves the reader. Your main goal is to convey your ideas with the greatest possible clarity. —Joseph Kimble[1]

A. The excerpt

This case study looks at an excerpt from an article published in *JAMA Internal Medicine*. The article tells about a study of 1,000 general medicine patients re-admitted within 30 days of discharge. Of these re-admissions, 269 were considered *preventable*, and the other 731 *non-preventable*. This excerpt describes factors associated with potentially preventable readmissions. Read the excerpt out loud:

> Multiple potential underlying <u>factors</u> <u>were</u> {<u>noted</u>} when we compared preventable and nonpreventable readmissions in the domains of med-ication safety, care coordination, discharge planning, advance care planning, promotion of self-management, enlisting of help and so-cial supports, diagnostic and therapeutic problems, and monitoring and managing of symptoms after discharge. Of potential underlying factors, those <u>variables</u> with the largest absolute differences in prev-alence between preventable and nonpreventable readmissions <u>were</u> the following: inadequate treatment of symptoms other than pain (20.8% [56 of 269] vs 6.4% [47 of 731]), inadequate monitoring for medication adverse effects or nonadherence (14.9% [40 of 269] vs 4.4% [32 of 731]), follow-up appointments not scheduled sufficiently soon after discharge (16.0% [43 of 269] vs 5.7% [42 of 731]), patient lack of awareness of whom to contact after discharge or when to go (or not to go) to the emergency department (18.6% [50 of 269] vs 5.7% [42 of 731]), patient need for additional or different home services than those services included in discharge plans (17.8% [48 of 269] vs 7.8% [57 of 731]), discharge of patients too soon (eg, symptoms such

as inability to eat or dyspnea not completely managed) from the index hospitalization (19.3% [52 of 269] vs 4.0% [29 of 731]), and issues related to the decision to admit the patient made in the emergency department (eg, the patient may not have required an inpatient stay, or useful information from the primary care physician was not available or reviewed) (12.6% [34 of 269] vs 2.6% [19 of 731]) (Table 4). *(WSEG = 252/126.0/0.0/57.5)*

Note: "Table 4," mentioned at the end of the excerpt, lists all of the potential underlying factors that lead to re-admissions, together with their related data. The factors are grouped by domain.

B. Analyzing the excerpt

1. Initial thoughts

What are some of your initial thoughts on this excerpt?
- *It uses many long words.*
- *It uses elegant variation—"variables" and "factors."*
- *It is written as one long paragraph.*
- *It contains many statistics written as prose.*
- *It uses very long sentences that include long lists.*

2. Looking at the WSEG score

a. Is the paragraph longer than 150 words? <u>*Yes*</u>. If so, do you see a good way to split it into shorter paragraphs?
   We could split the paragraph into two. One paragraph could talk about the "domains." The other could talk about the most important "factors" leading to preventable re-admissions.

b. How does this excerpt's average sentence length compare with the recommended average of 15 words?
   It has an average sentence length of 126 words—more than eight times the recommended average.

c. How many words does each sentence use? First <u>*47*</u>, second <u>*205*</u>

d. For each sentence that uses more than 25 words, do you think it needs to be just one long sentence? Why or why not?

Both of the excerpt's sentences use more than 25 words. They both contain lists. We could probably break them up into shorter sentences by organizing the lists differently and removing data duplicated in Table 4.

e. Does the reading ease score fall between 45 and 70 (the one standard deviation range)? <u>*No*</u>; or between 33 and 83 (the two standard deviation range)? <u>*No*</u>

f. Does the grade level fall between 6 and 11 (the one standard deviation range)? <u>*No*</u>; or between 4 and 13 (the two standard deviation range)? <u>*No*</u>

3. Looking at grammar

a. For each sentence in the excerpt, underline the <u>subject</u> and double underline the <u>main verb</u>. If the main verb includes a past participle, then draw braces around the {<u>past participle</u>}.

b. Fill in Table 10-1, answering the questions for each sentence.

Table 10-1. **Analyze the grammar of each sentence**

Sentence	Does the main verb contain a form of to be?	Is the sentence active, passive or neither?	Is the subject abstract or concrete?	Are the subject and verb close together in the first 7–8 words?
1st	yes	passive	abstract	yes
2nd	yes	neither	abstract	no

c. For each abstract subject, explain, in your own words, why it is abstract.
  - *"Factors" is a generalization about a class of activities that leads to re-admission.*
  - *"Variables" is used here as elegant variation for "factors."*

d. What words or ideas are written in the plural?

Factors, readmissions, domains, supports, problems, symptoms, variables, differences, effects, appointments, services, plans, patients, issues

e. What words or ideas need to be plural?

Factors, readmissions, symptoms, variables, effects, services, plans, patients, issues

f. Fill in Table 10-2 to show your thinking about any phrase that shows possession or connection using *of* or a word ending other than 's.

Table 10-2. **Revising phrases that show possession or connection using *of* or a word ending**

List the phrase, underlining *of* or the *word ending*	Is the possession or connection real world or abstract?	How might you replace *of* or the word ending?
domains *of* medic*ation* safety, care coordin*ation*	abstract	groups (*of* factors): medicine safety, coordinating care
promot*ion of* self-management	abstract	teach the patient how to take care *of* themself
enlisting *of* help and social supports	real world	finding help and social support
diagnos*tic* and therap*eutic* problems	abstract	problems with diagnosis and treatment
monitoring and managing *of* symptoms	abstract	monitoring and managing symptoms
inadequate treatment *of* symptoms	real world	symptoms not treated well enough
(20.8% [56 *of* 269] vs 6.4% [47 *of* 731])	abstract	(no change)
patient lack *of* awareness *of* whom to contact	abstract	patient doesn't know whom to contact
discharge *of* patients too soon	abstract	patient discharged too soon

4. Prefer the short word

a. Here is a fresh copy of the excerpt. Underline each <u>long word</u>.

<u>Multiple</u> <u>potential</u> <u>underlying</u> factors were noted when we compared <u>preventable</u> and <u>nonpreventable</u> <u>readmissions</u> in the domains of <u>medication</u> safety, care <u>coordination</u>, discharge planning, advance care planning, <u>promotion</u> of <u>self-management</u>, enlisting of help and social supports, <u>diagnostic</u> and <u>therapeutic</u> problems, and <u>monitoring</u> and managing of symptoms after discharge. Of <u>potential</u> <u>underlying</u> factors, those <u>variables</u> with the largest <u>absolute</u> <u>differences</u> in <u>prevalence</u> between <u>preventable</u> and <u>nonpreventable</u>

<u>readmissions</u> were the following: <u>inadequate</u> treatment of symptoms other than pain (20.8% [56 of 269] vs 6.4% [47 of 731]), <u>inadequate</u> <u>monitoring</u> for <u>medication</u> adverse effects or <u>nonadherence</u> (14.9% [40 of 269] vs 4.4% [32 of 731]), <u>follow-up</u> <u>appointments</u> not scheduled <u>sufficiently</u> soon after discharge (16.0% [43 of 269] vs 5.7% [42 of 731]), patient lack of <u>awareness</u> of whom to contact after discharge or when to go (or not to go) to the <u>emergency</u> <u>department</u> (18.6% [50 of 269] vs 5.7% [42 of 731]), patient need for <u>additional</u> or <u>different</u> home services than those services included in discharge plans (17.8% [48 of 269] vs 7.8% [57 of 731]), discharge of patients too soon (eg, symptoms such as <u>inability</u> to eat or <u>dyspnea</u> not <u>completely</u> managed) from the index <u>hospitalization</u> (19.3% [52 of 269] vs 4.0% [29 of 731]), and issues related to the <u>decision</u> to admit the patient made in the <u>emergency</u> <u>department</u> (eg, the patient may not have required an <u>inpatient</u> stay, or useful <u>information</u> from the <u>primary</u> care <u>physician</u> was not <u>available</u> or reviewed) (12.6% [34 of 269] vs 2.6% [19 of 731]) (Table 4).

b. Count the number of <u>long words</u> and compute long words as a percent of total words.
    <u>47</u> long words/252 total words = <u>18.7</u>%.
c. Double underline any <u>long word</u> you consider a <u>proper name</u> or <u>essential scientific term</u>.
d. For each <u>long word</u> you underlined just once (i.e., skip the essential scientific terms), fill in Table 10-3.

Table 10-3. **Finding shorter words**

Long word	Real world or abstract?	Shorter words that mean about the same thing
multiple	*abstract*	*many, a number, a few, some, more than one*
potential	*abstract*	*likely, possible, probable, may, could be*
underlying	*abstract*	*hidden, underneath, cause, important, beneath*
preventable	*abstract*	*prevent, able to prevent, able to stop, avoid, can prevent*
nonpreventable	*abstract*	*not preventable, could not prevent, not able to stop, can not avoid*
readmissions	*abstract*	*re-admit, admit again, back in hospital*
medication	*real world*	*medicine, drug, prescription*
coordination	*abstract*	*coordinate, agree, unite, same, consistent*

Long word	Real world or abstract?	Shorter words that mean about the same thing
promotion	abstract	promote, encourage, help, teach, allow, cause
self-management	real world	manage self, take care of oneself, do it themselves, at home, self-care
diagnostic	abstract	diagnose, figure out what is wrong
therapeutic	abstract	therapy, treatment, treat, treating
monitoring	abstract	monitor, keep track of, look out for, be aware of, look at, check on
variables	abstract	factors, vary, things
prevalence	abstract	number of, people with, rate, percent
inadequate	abstract	not adequate, not enough, wrong, bad, not the right (treatment)
nonadherence	abstract	not following doctor's orders, not taking drugs as prescribed, not doing
follow-up	abstract	next, check up, to follow up, later
appointments	real world	visit, see doctor, date
sufficiently	abstract	enough, good
awareness	abstract	be aware, knowledge, know
emergency department	real world	ER, emergency room, accident room
additional	abstract	other, another, more, also, too
different	abstract	other
inability	abstract	unable, not able, can't
dyspnea	real world	shortness of breath, short of breath, trouble breathing, can't breathe well, out of breath
completely	abstract	all, fully, wholly
hospitalization	real world	admitted, hospital visit, stay, inpatient stay, put in hospital
decision	abstract	choice, finding, decide, plan, thought
inpatient	abstract	admit
information	real world	facts, data, report, results, patient files
primary (care physician)	abstract	normal, usual, first, doctor, family doctor
physician	real world	doctor
available	abstract	there, at hand, on hand, reachable, handy, in the system, present, near, on file

e. Look at the long words listed in Table 10-3. Do any of them have the same or a similar meaning?

- *Multiple and additional*
- *Awareness and information*
- *Readmission, hospitalization and inpatient*
- *Follow-up and appointment*

f. Fill in Table 10-4 by listing each long word that is a nominalization and giving the root verb or adjective.

Table 10-4. **Find the root verb or adjective for each nominalization**

Nominalization	Root verb or adjective
readmissions	to (re)admit
medication	to medicate
coordination	to coordinate
promotion	to promote
self-management	to manage (self)
monitoring	to monitor
variable	to vary
prevalence	to prevail
nonadherence	to (not) adhere
follow-up	to follow up
appointments	to appoint
awareness	aware
inability	unable
hospitalization	to hospitalize
decision	to decide
information	to inform

g. Does the excerpt use any compound word(s) whose meaning or pronunciation might be clearer if hyphenated or written as an open compound? If so, tell which one(s) and why you think so.

We might hyphenate "non-preventable," "re-admissions," and "non-adherence," so people can better see the two parts.

5. Looking at meaning and logic

a. What is the issue or problem this excerpt deals with?
   Of the factors that lead to a patient being re-admitted to the hospital, which ones are most preventable?

b. With regard to this issue or problem, does the excerpt: describe it? tell why it is important? offer a solution?
   This excerpt offers a solution. It applies a math procedure to identify the seven top preventable factors.

c. Does the excerpt frame the issue or problem in real-world terms or abstract terms? Or does it only imply the issue or problem?
   The "factors" relate to real-world activities (e.g., medication safety, care coordination). The math procedure used to analyze the factors is abstract.

C. Prescription for revising

Write your prescription for revising to treat the symptoms of *medicus incomprehensibilis*. List the things you would recommend to help improve reading ease and clarity.

- *Omit the numerical data (which is repeated in Table 4 mentioned in the excerpt)*
- *Introduce and develop one idea in each paragraph*
- *Keep sentence length 15 words average, 25 words maximum*
- *Write in the singular*
- *Omit any unnecessary of*
- *Omit any unnecessary word ending*
- *Keep essential scientific terms; minimize other long words*
- *Convert nominalization into a verb in active voice*

D. Revision

Revise the excerpt to improve reading ease and clarity. In your revision, omit the numerical data (which is repeated in Table 4). Consider using tables, bullet points, or numbered lists in your revision.

What factors lead to a patient being <u>re-admitted</u> to the <u>hospital</u>?
We checked the charts for 1,000 patients who got <u>re-admitted</u> and noted the factors that led to their <u>re-admission</u>. We give data on each factor in Table 4. We found that these factors fell into eight groups (Table A).

Table A. **Groups of factors leading to _re-admissions_**

1. _Medicine_ safety	5. Teaching the patient to take care of themself
2. _Coordinating_ care	6. Finding help and social support
3. Discharge planning	7. Problem with _diagnosis_ or treatment
4. Advance care planning	8. _Monitoring_ and managing symptoms after discharge

Which _re-admissions_ could have been prevented?

We asked our panel of _reviewers_ to judge whether or not each _admission_ could have been prevented. They judged that 269 could have been prevented and 731 could not.

We then reviewed the data and tried to decide which factors were most _preventable_. This would help us know where to focus our efforts to improve. We decided the most _preventable_ factors were those with the biggest _absolute difference_ between the rates of _re-admissions_ that were _preventable_ and those that weren't. Table B shows the factors we selected.

Table B. **Factors leading to a patient being _re-admitted_ that seem most _preventable_**

1. Symptoms (other than pain) not treated well enough.
2. Not enough _monitoring_ for adverse effects or whether the patient took their _medicine_ as prescribed.
3. Patient _follow-up_ was scheduled for a time that was too long after discharge.
4. The patient didn't know whom to contact after discharge or when they should go to the ER.
5. The patient needed more or other home services than those included in the discharge plans.
6. The patient was discharged from the first stay too soon. (E.g., their symptoms such as "could not eat" or "trouble breathing" were not fully managed.)
7. Issues related to the ER's choice to _re-admit_ the patient. (E.g., the patient did not need to be _re-admitted_ to the _hospital_. Or else, useful data from the patient's _primary_ care doctor was not _available_ or not reviewed.)

1. Looking at WSEG scores

Compute the WSEG score for your revision. Fill in Table 10-5 to show how your revision compares with the original.

Table 10-5. **Comparing WSEG scores**

WSEG		Original	Revised	Change
W	Number of words	252	335	83
S	Average sentence length	126.0	13.3	−112.7
E	Flesch Reading Ease score	0.0	64.3	64.3
G	Flesch-Kincaid Grade Level	57.5	7.6	−49.9

2. Looking at grammar

Answer the following questions about your revision:

a. Does each sentence put the subject and verb close together within the first 7 or 8 words? If not, tell why it seemed best to do otherwise.
   In Table B, item 7, last sentence—the long logical subject prevents us from putting the subject, "data," and verb, "was," close together in the first 7 or 8 words.

b. Does each sentence use active voice? If not, tell why it seemed best to do otherwise.
   We had a few sentences that do not use active voice.
   • *The heading "Which re-admissions could have been prevented?" is passive. The important thing is, which re-admissions could have been prevented, not who could have prevented them.*
   • *Table B, items 3, 6, and 7 use passive voice. In each case, who did the action is not important.*

c. Does each sentence use a concrete subject? If not, tell why it seemed best to use an abstract subject.
   In our revision, we used mostly concrete subjects to explain what the researchers did. We isolated the abstract ideas, those issues that led to patients being re-admitted, in Tables A and B.

3. Prefer the short word

a. Underline each long word. Count the number of long words and compute long words as a percent of total words. 28 long words/335 total words = 8.4%. Compare your answer with the percent of long words in the original. (See §B.4.b.)

b. Double underline any long word you consider a proper name or essential scientific term.

4. Additional comments

Why did our revision use 83 more words than the original?
The original used long sentences that were difficult to follow. Each sentence had a long list; the items on each list consisted of whole phrases. Our revisions turned each sentence into a paragraph, and each phrase into its own sentence. We also tried to explain things in real-world terms that are easier to visualize and understand. This took more words, but became much clearer. Our effort to improve reading ease led to a big improvement in logical organization.

Note

1. Joseph Kimble, *Lifting the Fog of Legalese: Essays on Plain Language* (Durham, NC: Carolina Academic Press, 2006), 96.

11

Integrating Genetic Testing Results into Clinical Practice

Short paragraphs put air around what you write and make it look inviting, whereas one long chunk of type can discourage a reader from even starting to read. —William Zinsser, *On Writing Well: The Classic Guide to Writing Nonfiction*[1]

A. The excerpt

This case study looks at an excerpt from an article published in *The American Journal of Medicine.*[2] Read the excerpt out loud:

> Importantly, our data suggest a disconnect between patient expectations and actual clinical practice. Most of the RIGHT Protocol patients from a previous survey believed that their health care providers would use their pharmacogenomic information when prescribing medications; however, over half of the clinicians surveyed did not expect to use, or did not know whether they would use, pharmacogenomic information in the future. This disconnect is especially problematic for clinicians because patient perspectives on the use of genomic data for personalized care may be significantly influenced by the media and for-profit genetic testing companies, which can market directly to consumers. For example, recent articles in *The New York Times* highlight the "Promise of Genetic Testing in Medicine," while an additional on-line article highlights a partnership between Rite Aid pharmacies (Camp Hill, Pa.) and Harmonyx (Cordova, Tenn.), a genetic testing company, to offer a range of genetic tests directly to consumers. Such stories highlight the enthusiasm for use of genetic testing in clinical practice, but clinician engagement will be key to ensuring the genetic information is actually translated into clinical care. Patients typically do not have the background knowledge to fully interpret their genetic data, and independent companies marketing these tests are not typically integrated with health care systems. Direct-to-consumer pharmacogenomic testing has been associated with increases in physician utilization, because patients will bring genetic testing results to the attention of their health

care providers. However, our data indicate that clinician concerns about use of pharmacogenomic information may pose one possible stumbling block toward integration and use of genomic testing into care, and could prevent pharmacogenomic data from being fully utilized in clinical practice. (*WSEG* = 272/34.0/10.0/19.3)

Note: the *RIGHT Protocol* stands for the *Right Drug, Right Dose, Right Time Protocol*.

B. Analyzing the excerpt

1. Initial thoughts

What are some of your initial thoughts on this excerpt?

2. Looking at the *WSEG* score

a. Is the paragraph longer than 150 words? ____ If so, do you see a good way to split it into shorter paragraphs?

b. How does this excerpt's average sentence length compare with the recommended average sentence length of 15 words?

c. Count the number of words in each sentence. Then calculate the total number of words. Write your answers in Table 11-1.

Table 11-1. **Words per sentence**

	Sentence								
	1st	2nd	3rd	4th	5th	6th	7th	8th	Total
Number of words									

d. For each sentence that uses more than 25 words, do you think it needs to be just one long sentence? Why or why not?

e. Does the reading ease score fall between 45 and 70 (the one standard deviation range)? ___; or between 33 and 83 (the two standard deviation range)? ___

f. Does the grade level fall between 6 and 11 (the one standard deviation range)? ___; or between 4 and 13 (the two standard deviation range)? ___

3. Looking at grammar

a. For each sentence in the excerpt, underline the subject and double underline the main verb. If the main verb includes a past participle, then draw braces around the {past participle}.

b. Fill in Table 11-2, answering the questions for each sentence.

Table 11-2. **Analyze the grammar of each sentence**

Sentence	Does the main verb contain a form of to be?	Is the sentence active, passive or neither?	Is the subject abstract or concrete?	Are the subject and verb close together in the first 7–8 words?
1st				
2nd				
3rd				
4th				
5th				
6th				
7th				
8th				

c. For each abstract subject, explain, in your own words, why it is abstract.

d. What words or ideas are written in the plural?

e. What words or ideas need to be plural?

f. Fill in Table 11-3 to show your thinking about any phrase that shows possession or connection using *of* or a word ending other than *'s*.

Table 11-3. **Revising phrases that show possession or connection using *of* or a word ending**

List the phrase, underlining of or the word ending	Is the possession or connection real world or abstract?	How might you replace *of* or the word ending?

4. Prefer the short word

a. Here is a fresh copy of the excerpt. Underline each <u>long word</u>.

> Importantly, our data suggest a disconnect between patient expectations and actual clinical practice. Most of the RIGHT Protocol patients from a previous survey believed that their health care providers would use their pharmacogenomic information when prescribing medications; however, over half of the clinicians surveyed did not expect to use, or did not know whether they would use, pharmacogenomic information in the future. This disconnect is especially problematic for clinicians because patient perspectives on the use of genomic data for personalized care may be significantly influenced by the media and for-profit genetic testing companies, which can market directly to consumers. For example, recent articles in *The New York Times* highlight the "Promise of Genetic Testing

in Medicine," while an additional on-line article highlights a partnership between Rite Aid pharmacies (Camp Hill, Pa.) and Harmonyx (Cordova, Tenn.), a genetic testing company, to offer a range of genetic tests directly to consumers. Such stories highlight the enthusiasm for use of genetic testing in clinical practice, but clinician engagement will be key to ensuring the genetic information is actually translated into clinical care. Patients typically do not have the background knowledge to fully interpret their genetic data, and independent companies marketing these tests are not typically integrated with health care systems. Direct-to-consumer pharmacogenomic testing has been associated with increases in physician utilization, because patients will bring genetic testing results to the attention of their health care providers. However, our data indicate that clinician concerns about use of pharmacogenomic information may pose one possible stumbling block toward integration and use of genomic testing into care, and could prevent pharmacogenomic data from being fully utilized in clinical practice.

b. Count the number of <u>long words</u> and compute long words as a percent of total words.

____ long words/272 total words = ____ %.

c. Double underline any <u>long word</u> you consider a <u>proper name</u> or <u>essential scientific term</u>.

d. For each <u>long word</u> you underlined just once (i.e., skip the essential scientific terms), fill in Table 11-4.

Table 11-4. **Finding shorter words**

Long word	Real world or abstract?	Shorter words that mean about the same thing

Long word	Real world or abstract?	Shorter words that mean about the same thing

Long word	Real world or abstract?	Shorter words that mean about the same thing

e. Look at the long words listed in Table 11-4. Do any of them have the same or a similar meaning?

f. Fill in Table 11-5 by listing each long word that is a nominalization and giving the root verb or adjective.

Table 11-5. **Find the root verb or adjective for each nominalization**

Nominalization	Root verb or adjective

g. Does the excerpt use any compound word(s) whose meaning or pronunciation might be clearer if hyphenated or written as an open compound? If so, tell which one(s) and why you think so.

5. Looking at meaning and logic

a. What is the issue or problem this excerpt deals with?

b. With regard to this issue or problem, does the excerpt: describe it? tell why it is important? offer a solution?

c. Does the excerpt frame the issue or problem in real-world terms or abstract terms? Or does it only imply the issue or problem?

C. Prescription for revising

Write your prescription for revising to treat the symptoms of *medicus incomprehensibilis*. List the things you would recommend to help improve reading ease and clarity.

D. Revision

Revise the excerpt to improve reading ease and clarity.

1. Looking at *WSEG* scores

Compute the *WSEG* score for your revision. Fill in Table 11-6 to show how your revision compares with the original.

Table 11-6. **Comparing *WSEG* scores**

WSEG		*Original*	*Revised*	*Change*
W	Number of words	272		
S	Average sentence length	34.0		
E	Flesch Reading Ease score	10.0		
G	Flesch-Kincaid Grade Level	19.3		

2. Looking at grammar

Answer the following questions about your revision:

a. Does each sentence put the subject and verb close together within the first 7 or 8 words? If not, tell why it seemed best to do otherwise.

b. Does each sentence use active voice? If not, tell why it seemed best to do otherwise.

c. Does each sentence use a concrete subject? If not, tell why it seemed best to use an abstract subject.

3. Prefer the short word

a. Underline each <u>long word</u>. Count the number of long words and compute long words as a percent of total words. ___ long words / ___ total words = ___ %. Compare your answer with the percent of long words in the original. (See §B.4.b.)

b. Double underline any <u>long word</u> you consider a <u>proper name</u> or <u>essential scientific term</u>.

Notes

1. William Zinsser, *On Writing Well: The Classic Guide to Writing*, 30th anniversary ed. (New York: Collins, 2006), 79.
2. Jennifer St. Sauver et al., "Integrating Pharmacogenomics into Clinical Practice: Promise vs Reality," *Am J Med* 129, no. 10 (October 2016): 1097.

Integrating Genetic Testing Results into Clinical Practice

Writers of plain English let their audience concentrate on the message instead of being distracted by complicated language. —Baden Eunson[1]

A. The excerpt

This case study looks at an excerpt from an article published in *The American Journal of Medicine*. Read the excerpt out loud:

> Importantly, our <u>data</u> <u>suggest</u> a disconnect between patient expectations and actual clinical practice. <u>Most</u> of the RIGHT Protocol patients from a previous survey <u>believed</u> that their health care providers would use their pharmacogenomic information when prescribing medications; however, over half of the clinicians surveyed did not expect to use, or did not know whether they would use, pharmacogenomic information in the future. This <u>disconnect</u> <u>is</u> especially problematic for clinicians because patient perspectives on the use of genomic data for personalized care may be significantly influenced by the media and for-profit genetic testing companies, which can market directly to consumers. For example, recent <u>articles</u> in *The New York Times* <u>highlight</u> the "Promise of Genetic Testing in Medicine," while an additional on-line article highlights a partnership between Rite Aid pharmacies (Camp Hill, Pa.) and Harmonyx (Cordova, Tenn.), a genetic testing company, to offer a range of genetic tests directly to consumers. Such <u>stories</u> <u>highlight</u> the enthusiasm for use of genetic testing in clinical practice, but clinician engagement will be key to ensuring the genetic information is actually translated into clinical care. <u>Patients</u> typically <u>do not have</u> the background knowledge to fully interpret their genetic data, and independent companies marketing these tests are not typically integrated with health care systems. Direct-to-consumer pharmacogenomic <u>testing has been {associated}</u> with increases in physician utilization, because patients will bring genetic testing results to the attention of their health

care providers. However, our <u>data indicate</u> that clinician concerns about use of pharmacogenomic information may pose one possible stumbling block toward integration and use of genomic testing into care, and could prevent pharmacogenomic data from being fully utilized in clinical practice. (*WSEG = 272/34.0/10.0/19.3*)

Note: the *RIGHT Protocol* stands for the *Right Drug, Right Dose, Right Time Protocol.*

B. Analyzing the excerpt

1. Initial thoughts

What are some of your initial thoughts on this excerpt?
- *A few sentences seem to cover multiple ideas.*
- *Some sentences are very long.*
- *It uses elegant variation: pharmacogenomic information, genomic data, genetic testing, genetic tests, genetic information, genetic data, pharmacogenomic testing, genomic testing, and pharmacogenomic data.*

2. Looking at the WSEG score

a. Is the paragraph longer than 150 words? <u>*Yes*</u>. If so, do you see a good way to split it into shorter paragraphs?
   We could split this long paragraph into three shorter paragraphs that tell: What is the disconnect? Why is this disconnect a problem for clinicians? and Why is clinician engagement and integration important?

b. How does this excerpt's average sentence length compare with the recommended average sentence length of 15 words?
   It has an average sentence length of 34.0 words—more than twice the recommended average.

c. Count the number of words in each sentence. Then calculate the total number of words. Write your answers in Table 11-1.

Table 11-1. **Words per sentence**

	Sentence								
	1st	*2nd*	*3rd*	*4th*	*5th*	*6th*	*7th*	*8th*	*Total*
Number of words	*13*	*49*	*37*	*50*	*30*	*28*	*26*	*39*	*272*

d. For each sentence that uses more than 25 words, do you think it needs to be just one long sentence? Why or why not?
   All sentences but the first use more than 25 words. Most can be broken up into shorter sentences.
   - *Second sentence—We could separate the two independent clauses with a period, instead of a semi-colon.*
   - *Third sentence—We could say, in one sentence, that the disconnect is a problem. Then, in another sentence, we can tell why.*
   - *Fourth sentence—We could talk about the recent articles on the "Promise of Genetic Testing in Medicine" in one sentence. Then, in another sentence, we could talk about the article on the partnership between Rite Aid pharmacies and Harmonyx.*
   - *Fifth sentence—We could talk about the enthusiasm in one sentence. Then, in another sentence, we could talk about clinical engagement.*
   - *Sixth sentence— In one sentence, we could talk about how patients don't have the background knowledge to interpret their own genetic data. Then, in another sentence, we could talk about how genetic testing companies are not integrated with health care systems.*
   - *Seventh sentence—We could talk about the increase in physician utilization in one sentence. Then, in another sentence, we could explain that the increase was due to patients bringing their results with them to the doctor.*
   - *Eighth sentence—Seems redundant; we would condense.*

e. Does the reading ease score fall between 45 and 70 (the one standard deviation range)? <u>*No*</u>; or between 33 and 83 (the two standard deviation range)? <u>*No*</u>

f. Does the grade level fall between 6 and 11 (the one standard deviation range)? <u>*No*</u>; or between 4 and 13 (the two standard deviation range)? <u>*No*</u>

3. Looking at grammar

a. For each sentence in the excerpt, underline the <u>subject</u> and double underline the <u>main verb</u>. If the main verb includes a past participle, then draw braces around the {<u>past participle</u>}.

b. Fill in Table 11-2, answering the questions for each sentence.

Table 11-2. **Analyze the grammar of each sentence**

Sentence	Does the main verb contain a form of *to be*?	Is the sentence active, passive or neither?	Is the subject abstract or concrete?	Are the subject and verb close together in the first 7–8 words?
1st	no	active	abstract	yes
2nd	no	active	abstract	no
3rd	yes	neither	abstract	yes
4th	no	active	abstract	no
5th	no	active	abstract	yes
6th	no	active	concrete	yes
7th	yes	passive	abstract	yes
8th	no	active	abstract	yes

c. For each abstract subject, explain, in your own words, why it is abstract.
  - "Data" refers to information.
  - "Most" refers to an assessment of a group of patients.
  - "Disconnect" refers to the difference between how the patient thinks their doctor decides what to prescribe and how the doctor actually decides.
  - "Articles/stories" refers to the ideas within the articles, not the physical pieces of paper.
  - "Testing" refers to the whole testing process, not just the physical objects used to conduct the test.

d. What words or ideas are written in the plural?
  Expectations, patients, providers, medications, clinicians, perspectives, companies, consumers, Times, articles, pharmacies, tests, stories, systems, increases, results, concerns

e. What words or ideas need to be plural?
  Patients, providers, clinicians, companies, articles, Times, pharmacies, tests, stories, results

f. Fill in Table 11-3 to show your thinking about any phrase that shows possession or connection using *of* or a word ending other than *'s*.

Table 11-3. **Revising phrases that show possession or connection using *of* or a word ending**

List the phrase, underlining *of* or the <u>word ending</u>	Is the possession or connection real world or abstract?	How might you replace of or the word ending?
most <u>of</u> the RIGHT Protocol patients	abstract	most RIGHT Protocol patients
pharmacogenom<u>ic</u> information	abstract	(no change)
half <u>of</u> the clinicians	abstract	(no change)
use <u>of</u> genom<u>ic</u> data	abstract	use gen<u>etic</u> data
Promise <u>of</u> Gen<u>etic</u> Testing in Medicine	abstract	(no change—quote)
range <u>of</u> gen<u>etic</u> tests	abstract	several gen<u>etic</u> tests
use <u>of</u> gen<u>etic</u> testing	abstract	using gen<u>etic</u> testing
bring [. . .] to the attention <u>of</u> their health care providers	abstract	show/tell their doctor
use <u>of</u> pharmacogenom<u>ic</u> information	abstract	using test results
use <u>of</u> genom<u>ic</u> testing	abstract	using gen<u>etic</u> test results

4. Prefer the short word

a. Here is a fresh copy of the excerpt. Underline each <u>long word</u>.

<u>Importantly</u>, our data suggest a <u>disconnect</u> between patient <u>expectations</u> and <u>actual</u> <u>clinical</u> practice. Most of the RIGHT <u>Protocol</u> patients from a <u>previous</u> survey believed that their health care <u>providers</u> would use their <u>pharmacogenomic</u> <u>information</u> when prescribing <u>medications</u>; <u>however</u>, over half of the <u>clinicians</u> surveyed did not expect to use, or did not know whether they would use, <u>pharmacogenomic</u> <u>information</u> in the future. This <u>disconnect</u> is <u>especially</u> <u>problematic</u> for <u>clinicians</u> because patient <u>perspectives</u> on the use of <u>genomic</u> data for <u>personalized</u> care may be <u>significantly</u> <u>influenced</u> by

the media and for-profit genetic testing companies, which can market directly to consumers. For example, recent articles in *The New York Times* highlight the "Promise of Genetic Testing in Medicine," while an additional on-line article highlights a partnership between Rite Aid pharmacies (Camp Hill, Pa.) and Harmonyx (Cordova, Tenn.), a genetic testing company, to offer a range of genetic tests directly to consumers. Such stories highlight the enthusiasm for use of genetic testing in clinical practice, but clinician engagement will be key to ensuring the genetic information is actually translated into clinical care. Patients typically do not have the background knowledge to fully interpret their genetic data, and independent companies marketing these tests are not typically integrated with health care systems. Direct-to-consumer pharmacogenomic testing has been associated with increases in physician utilization, because patients will bring genetic testing results to the attention of their health care providers. However, our data indicate that clinician concerns about use of pharmacogenomic information may pose one possible stumbling block toward integration and use of genomic testing into care, and could prevent pharmacogenomic data from being fully utilized in clinical practice.

b. Count the number of long words and compute long words as a percent of total words.

80 long words/272 total words = 29.4%.

c. Double underline any long word you consider a proper name or essential scientific term.

d. For each long word you underlined just once (i.e., skip the essential scientific terms), fill in Table 11-4.

Table 11-4. **Finding shorter words**

Long word	Real world or abstract?	Shorter words that mean about the same thing
importantly	*abstract*	*notably, important, key*
disconnect	*abstract*	*gap, divide, differ*
expectations	*abstract*	*thought, idea, wish, want, desire, expect*
actual	*abstract*	*real, what happens, true, current, in fact*
clinical	*abstract?*	*in practice, treating a patient, clinic*
previous	*abstract*	*past, other, before, early, former*

Long word	Real world or abstract?	Shorter words that mean about the same thing
providers	real world	doctor, nurse, hospital, clinic
pharmacogenomic	real world	gene, gene response to a drug, genetic test, gene test, genetic information, genetic data
information	abstract	facts, data, report, results, test results
medications	real world	medicine, drug, pill, shot
however	abstract	but, yet, in spite of, despite
clinicians	real world	doctor, nurse, dentist
especially	abstract	big, major, notable, very, more so, even more, really
problematic	abstract	problem, issue, tricky, bad, worrisome, hard
perspectives	abstract	view, thought, idea, want, desire
genomic	real world?	genome, gene, genetic, genetic test
personalized	abstract	personal, person, their, for the patient, the patient's, unique, special, direct
significantly	abstract	greatly, very, major, big, much, noticeable, significant, really
influenced	abstract	guide, inform, convince
media	abstract	press, news, TV
for-profit	abstract	for profit, make money
genetic	real world?	gene, gene test
companies	real world?	firm
directly	abstract	direct, to, right to, without the doctor
consumers	real world	patient, people, user, person
example	abstract	e.g.
articles	abstract?	story, news item, piece, series, work
additional	abstract	other, another, more, also
partnership	abstract	link, deal, partner, pair, group, bond
pharmacies	real world	drug store, store
enthusiasm	abstract	desire, want, good feeling, joy, pleasure, excitement, excite, push, interest

Long word	Real world or abstract?	Shorter words that mean about the same thing
engagement	abstract	use, engage, involve, take part
actually	abstract	really, in fact, indeed, actual
typically	abstract	often, mainly, most, common, typical, type
interpret	abstract	read, know how to use, explain, give meaning to, decode, expound
independent	abstract	not dependent, not connected, separate, alone, not related, free
integrated	abstract	a part of, connect, together, link, join, tie to, talk to, share data
direct-to-consumer	abstract	direct to the consumer, straight to the patient, store bought, at home
associated	abstract	link to, paired, leads to, related, connected, causes
physician	real world	doctor
utilization	abstract	use, implement, take into account, read the test results
attention	abstract	to mind, make aware, tell, show
indicate	abstract	show, make clear, point out, suggest
possible	abstract	likely, maybe, can
integration	abstract	integrate, part of, connect, link, share data
utilized	abstract	use

e. Look at the long words listed in Table 11-4. Do any of them have the same or a similar meaning?

- *Importantly, especially and significantly*
- *Expectations and perspectives*
- *Pharmacogenomic, genomic and genetic*
- *Providers, clinician and physician*
- *Especially, significantly and typically*
- *Perspectives and attention*
- *Partnership, engagement and associated*
- *Integrated and integration*

f. Fill in Table 11-5 by listing each long word that is a nominalization and giving the root verb or adjective.

Table 11-5. **Find the root verb or adjective for each nominalization**

Nominalization	Root verb or adjective
disconnect	to (dis-) connect
expectations	to expect
providers	to provide
information	to inform
medications	to medicate
perspective	to perceive
consumers	to consume
partnership	to partner
engagement	to engage
utilization	to utilize, to use
attention	to attend to
integration	to integrate, integral

g. Does the excerpt use any compound word(s) whose meaning or pronunciation might be clearer if hyphenated or written as an open compound? If so, tell which one(s) and why you think so.
We might hyphenate "pharmaco-genomics" so people can better see the two parts.

5. Looking at meaning and logic

a. What is the issue or problem this excerpt deals with?
There is a gap in expectations. Patients tend to think their doctor will use their genetic data when prescribing medicine. The doctors tend to think differently.

b. With regard to this issue or problem, does the excerpt: describe it? tell why it is important? offer a solution?
The excerpt describes the problem and tells why it is important.

c. Does the excerpt frame the issue or problem in real-world terms or abstract terms? Or does it only imply the issue or problem?
This issue is abstract because it deals with how people think (but, it avoids sounding too abstract by talking about "patients" and "clinicians").

C. Prescription for revising

Write your prescription for revising to treat the symptoms of *medicus incomprehensibilis*. List the things you would recommend to help improve reading ease and clarity.

- *Introduce and develop one idea in each paragraph*
- *Keep sentence length 15 words average, 25 words maximum*
- *Keep the subject and verb close together in the first 7 or 8 words*
- *Put the main point first, then give commentary, detail or support*
- *Revise abstract into concrete*
- *Observe the 1066 principle*
- *Write in the singular*
- *Talk in terms of one doctor treating one patient*
- *Avoid using a high percentage of long words*
- *Keep essential scientific terms; minimize other long words*
- *Use terms consistently; avoid elegant variation*
- *Convert nominalization into a verb in active voice*

D. Revision

Revise the excerpt to improve reading ease and clarity.

> *Our data show a gap between what a patient expects and what happens in <u>clinical</u> practice. We know from a past survey that most of the RIGHT <u>Protocol</u> patients thought their doctor would use their <u>genetic</u> testing results when prescribing <u>medicine</u>. But over half of the doctors did not expect to use these results. Nor did they know if they would use them in the future.*
>
> *This gap may present a big problem for doctors. A patient's ideas on the use of <u>genetic</u> testing for health care may be guided by the media and <u>for-profit</u> <u>genetic</u> testing firms, which can market <u>directly</u> to the patient. For example, recent articles in The New York Times highlight the "Promise of <u>Genetic</u> Testing in <u>Medicine</u>." Another on-line article highlights a link between Rite Aid drug stores (Camp Hill, Pa.) and <u>Harmonyx</u> (<u>Cordova</u>, Tenn.), a <u>genetic</u> testing firm. Together, they offer a wide range of <u>genetic</u> tests direct to the patient.*
>
> *Stories like this highlight the public's desire for using <u>genetic</u> testing results in <u>clinical</u> practice. But involving the doctor will be key to ensuring the results get used in patient care. Most patients do not know how to use their <u>genetic</u> testing results. The firms that sell these tests are not often connected with a health care system. <u>Genetic</u> testing sold directly to the patient leads to the doctor using the test results more often, since a patient brings them to the doctor. But our data show that a doctor's concerns about using these test results may keep them from being used fully in practice.*

1. Looking at WSEG scores

Compute the WSEG score for your revision. Fill in Table 11-6 to show how your revision compares with the original.

Table 11-6. **Comparing WSEG scores**

WSEG		*Original*	*Revised*	*Change*
W	Number of words	272	262	–10
S	Average sentence length	34.0	17.4	–16.6
E	Flesch Reading Ease score	10.0	63.4	53.4
G	Flesch-Kincaid Grade Level	19.3	8.7	–10.6

2. Looking at grammar

Answer the following questions about your revision:

a. Does each sentence put the subject and verb close together within the first 7 or 8 words? If not, tell why it seemed best to do otherwise.
   - *In Paragraph 1, third sentence, the subject, "doctors," and the verb, "did not expect to use," are close together, but they don't come in the first 7 or 8 words.*
   - *In Paragraph 2, second sentence, the subject, "ideas," and verb, "may be guided," are separated by an explanation of the ideas.*
   - *In Paragraph 2, third sentence, the subject, "articles," and verb, "highlights," are separated by "in The New York Times."*
   - *In Paragraph 3, fourth sentence, the subject, "firms," and verb, "are not often connected," are separated by a description of the firms.*
   - *In Paragraph 4, first sentence, the subject, "testing," and verb, "leads," are separated by the phrase, "sold directly to the patient."*
b. Does each sentence use active voice? If not, tell why it seemed best to do otherwise.
   No.
   - *In Paragraph 2, the second sentence is passive. This tracks the original.*
   - *In Paragraph 3, the second and fourth sentences are both passive. This tracks the original.*
c. Does each sentence use a concrete subject? If not, tell why it seemed best to use an abstract subject.
   No, we used a number of abstract subjects (e.g., data, gap, ideas, articles, testing). These abstract subjects seemed appropriate, since the excerpt deals with generalizations about data and compares patients' and doctor's perspectives.

3. Prefer the short word

a. Underline each <u>long word</u>. Count the number of long words and compute long words as a percent of total words. <u>18</u> long words/<u>262</u> total words = <u>6.9</u>%. Compare your answer with the percent of long words in the original. (See §B.4.b.)

b. Double underline any <u>long word</u> you consider a <u>proper name</u> or <u>essential scientific term</u>.

Note

1. Baden Eunson, quoted in Primary Health Care Research & Information Service, "Introduction to Plain Language," http://www.phcris.org.au/guides/plain_language.php (accessed January 3, 2018).

How Tamoxifen Interacts with SSRI Anti-Depressants

Writing that is clear and to the point helps improve communication and takes less time to read and understand. Clear writing tells the reader exactly what the reader needs to know without using unnecessary words or expressions. —National Institutes of Health (USA)[1]

A. The excerpt

This case study looks at an excerpt from an editorial published in *The BMJ (British Medical Journal)*.[2] Read the excerpt out loud:

> Why does the interaction between tamoxifen and SSRIs remain controversial? One reason is that tamoxifen's pharmacokinetic fate involves processes other than CYP2D6. Another is that studies of the relation between CYP2D6 activity and outcomes in women receiving tamoxifen yield remarkably inconsistent results. Finally, with some exceptions, observational studies show little evidence that use of antidepressants is associated with adverse outcomes in women receiving tamoxifen.
>
> Donneyong and colleagues used data from five US health insurance databases to study women already being treated with an SSRI at the outset of treatment with tamoxifen or who received an SSRI later during its course. Over a median follow-up of about two years, they found no difference in overall mortality among women receiving SSRIs that inhibit CYP2D6 (paroxetine and fluoxetine) relative to SSRIs that do not (citalopram, escitalopram, fluvoxamine and sertraline).
>
> These findings are unsurprising, if for no other reason than follow-up was too brief for any differential survival to show up. Studying total mortality rather than cancer specific outcomes further diminished the investigators' ability to discern signal from noise. Consequently, this study does little to disprove a meaningful interaction between tamoxifen and CYP2D6 inhibitors. It does, however, illustrate just how challenging such studies can be.

Pharmacoepidemiology is a relative newcomer to the science of drug interactions, with most studies exploring short term toxicities after the co-prescription of drugs with well established interactions. In contrast, the interaction between tamoxifen and CYP2D6 inhibiting SSRIs is characterized by an elusive outcome (treatment failure), a long latent period, and many other factors (including non-adherence, therapeutic switching, CYP2D6 polymorphisms, dose-response effects, variable mechanisms and degrees of inhibition, and a probable endoxifen threshold below which treatment failure is more likely) that collectively attenuate any signal that might exist. For these reasons, the tamoxifen-SSRI interaction is perhaps the most difficult drug interaction to explore using the techniques of pharmacoepidemiology. (*WSEG = 308/23.6/10.8/17.6*)

Notes:

1. *Tamoxifen* is an estrogen receptor modulating drug used to treat breast cancer. It reduces the risk of recurrence of breast cancer in women with hormone re-ceptor positive tumors. Tamoxifen takes effect when it is metabolized, by means of the CYP2D6 enzyme, and converted into endoxifen.

2. *SSRI* stands for *selective serotonin reuptake inhibitor.* SSRIs are a class of drugs used to treat depression. Some SSRIs keep the body from producing the CYP2D6 enzyme.

3. Half of all women with breast cancer feel depressed or anxious in the first year after their diagnosis. One out of four women who take tamoxifen also take an SSRI.[3]

B. Analyzing the excerpt

1. Initial thoughts

What are some of your initial thoughts on this excerpt?

2. Looking at the *WSEG* score

a. How does this excerpt's average sentence length compare with the recommended average of 15 words?

b. Count the number of words in each sentence. Then calculate the total number of words for each paragraph. Write your answers in Table 12-1.

Table 12-1. **Words per sentence**

				Sentence				
	1st	2nd	3rd	4th	5th	6th	7th	Total
Paragraph 1					—	—	—	
Paragraph 2			—	—	—	—	—	
Paragraph 3								
Grand Total								

c. Is any paragraph longer than 150 words? ___ If so, do you see a good way to split it into shorter paragraphs?

d. For each sentence that uses more than 25 words, do you think it needs to be just one long sentence? Why or why not?

e. Does the reading ease score fall between 45 and 70 (the one standard deviation range)?___; or between 33 and 83 (the two standard deviation range)? ___

f. Does the grade level fall between 6 and 11 (the one standard deviation range)? ___; or between 4 and 13 (the two standard deviation range)? ___

3. Looking at grammar

a. For each sentence in the excerpt, underline the subject and double underline the main verb. If the main verb includes a past participle, then draw braces around the {past participle}.

b. Fill in Table 12-2, answering the questions for each sentence.

Table 12-2. **Analyze the grammar of each sentence**

Sentence	Does the main verb contain a form of to be?	Is the sentence active, passive or neither?	Is the subject abstract or concrete?	Are the subject and verb close together in the first 7–8 words?
Paragraph 1				
1st				
2nd				
3rd				
4th				
Paragraph 2				
1st				
2nd				
Paragraph 3				
1st				
2nd				
3rd				
4th				
5th				
6th				
7th				

c. For each abstract subject, explain, in your own words, why it is abstract.

d. What words or ideas are written in the plural?

e. What words or ideas need to be plural?

f. Fill in Table 12-3 to show your thinking about any phrase that shows possession or connection using *of* or a word ending other than *'s*.

Table 12-3. **Revising phrases that show possession or connection using *of* or a word ending**

List the phrase, underlining *of* or the <u>word ending</u>	Is the possession or connection real world or abstract?	How might you replace of or the word ending?

4. Prefer the short word

a. Here is a fresh copy of the excerpt. Underline each <u>long word</u>.

> Why does the interaction between tamoxifen and SSRIs remain controversial? One reason is that tamoxifen's pharmacokinetic fate involves processes other than CYP2D6. Another is that studies of the relation between CYP2D6 activity and outcomes in women receiving tamoxifen yield remarkably inconsistent results. Finally, with some exceptions, observational studies show little evidence that use of antidepressants is associated with adverse outcomes in women receiving tamoxifen.
>
> Donneyong and colleagues used data from five US health insurance databases to study women already being treated with an SSRI at the outset of treatment with tamoxifen or who received an SSRI later during its course. Over a median follow-up of about two years, they found no difference in overall mortality among women receiving SSRIs that inhibit CYP2D6 (paroxetine and fluoxetine) relative to SSRIs that do not (citalopram, escitalopram, fluvoxamine and sertraline).
>
> These findings are unsurprising, if for no other reason than follow-up was too brief for any differential survival to show up. Studying total mortality rather than cancer specific outcomes further diminished the investigators' ability to discern signal from noise. Consequently, this study does little to disprove a meaningful interaction between tamoxifen and CYP2D6 inhibitors. It does, however, illustrate just how challenging such studies can be. Pharmacoepidemiology is a relative newcomer to the science of drug interactions, with most studies exploring short term toxicities after the co-prescription of drugs with well established interactions. In contrast, the interaction between tamoxifen and CYP2D6 inhibiting SSRIs is characterized by an elusive outcome (treatment failure), a long latent period, and many other factors (including non-adherence, therapeutic switching, CYP2D6 polymorphisms, dose-response effects, variable mechanisms and degrees of inhibition, and a probable endoxifen threshold below which treatment failure is more likely) that collectively attenuate any signal that might exist. For these reasons, the tamoxifen-SSRI interaction is perhaps the most difficult drug interaction to explore using the techniques of pharmacoepidemiology.

b. Count the number of <u>long words</u> and compute long words as a percent of total words.

   ___ long words/308 total words = ___ %.

c. Double underline any <u>long word</u> you consider a <u>proper name</u> or <u>essential scientific term</u>.

d. For each <u>long word</u> you underlined just once (i.e., skip the essential scientific terms), fill in Table 12-4.

Table 12-4. **Finding shorter words**

Long word	Real world or abstract?	Shorter words that mean about the same thing

Long word	Real world or abstract?	Shorter words that mean about the same thing

Long word	Real world or abstract?	Shorter words that mean about the same thing

e. Look at the long words listed in Table 12-4. Do any of them have the same or a similar meaning?

f. Fill in Table 12-5 by listing each long word that is a nominalization and giving the root verb or adjective.

Table 12-5. **Find the root verb or adjective for each nominalization**

Nominalization	Root verb or adjective

Nominalization	*Root verb or adjective*

g. Does the excerpt use any compound word(s) whose meaning or pronunciation might be clearer if hyphenated or written as an open compound? If so, tell which one(s) and why you think so.

5. Looking at meaning and logic

a. What is the issue or problem this excerpt deals with?

b. With regard to this issue or problem, does the excerpt: describe it? tell why it is important? offer a solution?

c. Does the excerpt frame the issue or problem in real-world terms or abstract terms? Or does it only imply the issue or problem?

C. Prescription for revising

Write your prescription for revising to treat the symptoms of *medicus incomprehensibilis*. List the things you would recommend to help improve reading ease and clarity.

D. Revision

Revise the excerpt to improve reading ease and clarity.

1. Looking at WSEG scores

Compute the WSEG score for your revision. Fill in Table 12-6 to show how your revision compares with the original.

Table 12-6. **Comparing WSEG scores**

WSEG		Original	Revised	Change
W	Number of words	308		
S	Average sentence length	23.6		
E	Flesch Reading Ease score	10.8		
G	Flesch-Kincaid Grade Level	17.6		

2. Looking at grammar

Answer the following questions about your revision:

a. Does each sentence put the subject and verb close together within the first 7 or 8 words? If not, tell why it seemed best to do otherwise.

b. Does each sentence use active voice? If not, tell why it seemed best to do otherwise.

c. Does each sentence use a concrete subject? If not, tell why it seemed best to use an abstract subject.

3. Prefer the short word

a. Underline each <u>long word</u>. Count the number of long words and compute long words as a percent of total words. ___ long words / ___ total words = ___ %. Compare your answer with the percent of long words in the original. (See §B.4.b.)

b. Double underline any <u>long word</u> you consider a <u>proper name</u> or <u>essential scientific term</u>.

Notes

1. National Institutes of Health, "Plain Language at NIH," https://www.nih.gov/institutes-nih/nih-office-director/office-communications-public-liaison/clear-communication/plain-language (accessed February 5, 2018).
2. David Juurlink, "Revisiting the Drug Interaction between Tamoxifen and SSRI Antidepressants," *BMJ* 354, no. 8072 (September 2016), https://www.bmj.com/content/354/bmj.i5309.
3. Macarius Donneyong et al., "Risk of Mortality with Concomitant Use of Tamoxifen and Selective Serotonin Reuptake Inhibitors: Multi-database Cohort Study," *BMJ* 354, no. 8072 (September 2016), under "Introduction," https://www.bmj.com/content/354/bmj.i5014.

How Tamoxifen Interacts with SSRI Anti-Depressants

There is no great writing, only great rewriting. —Justice Louis Brandeis[1]

A. The excerpt

This case study looks at an excerpt from an editorial published in *The BMJ* *(British Medical Journal)*. Read the excerpt out loud:

Why <u>does</u> the <u>interaction</u> between tamoxifen and SSRIs <u>remain</u> controversial? One <u>reason</u> <u>is</u> that tamoxifen's pharmacokinetic fate involves processes other than CYP2D6. <u>Another</u> <u>is</u> that studies of the relation between CYP2D6 activity and outcomes in women receiving tamoxifen yield remarkably inconsistent results. Finally, with some exceptions, observational <u>studies</u> <u>show</u> little evidence that use of antidepressants is associated with adverse outcomes in women receiving tamoxifen.

<u>Donneyong and colleagues</u> <u>used</u> data from five US health insurance databases to study women already being treated with an SSRI at the outset of treatment with tamoxifen or who received an SSRI later during its course. Over a median follow-up of about two years, <u>they</u> <u>found</u> no difference in overall mortality among women receiving SSRIs that inhibit CYP2D6 (paroxetine and fluoxetine) relative to SSRIs that do not (citalopram, escitalopram, fluvoxamine and sertraline).

These <u>findings</u> <u>are</u> unsurprising, if for no other reason than follow-up was too brief for any differential survival to show up. <u>Studying</u> total mortality rather than cancer specific outcomes further <u>diminished</u> the investigators' ability to discern signal from noise. Consequently, this <u>study</u> <u>does</u> little to disprove a meaningful interaction between tamoxifen and CYP2D6 inhibitors. <u>It</u> <u>does</u>, however, <u>illustrate</u> just how challenging such studies can be. <u>Pharmacoepidemiology</u> <u>is</u> a relative newcomer to the science of drug interactions, with most studies exploring short term toxicities after the co-prescription of drugs with

well established interactions. In contrast, the <u>interaction</u> between tamoxifen and CYP2D6 inhibiting SSRIs <u>is</u> {<u>characterized</u>} by an elusive outcome (treatment failure), a long latent period, and many other
factors (including non-adherence, therapeutic switching, CYP2D6
polymorphisms, dose-response effects, variable mechanisms and
degrees of inhibition, and a probable endoxifen threshold below which
treatment failure is more likely) that collectively attenuate any signal
that might exist. For these reasons, the tamoxifen-SSRI <u>interaction</u>
<u>is</u> perhaps the most difficult drug interaction to explore using the
techniques of pharmacoepidemiology. (*WSEG = 308/23.6/10.8/17.6*)

Notes:
1. *Tamoxifen* is an estrogen receptor modulating drug used to treat breast cancer.
   It reduces the risk of recurrence of breast cancer in women with hormone receptor positive tumors. Tamoxifen takes effect when it is metabolized, by
   means of the CYP2D6 enzyme, and converted into endoxifen.
2. *SSRI* stands for *selective serotonin reuptake inhibitor*. SSRIs are a class of drugs
   used to treat depression. SSRIs tend to keep the body from producing the
   CYP2D6 enzyme.
3. Half of all women with breast cancer feel depressed or anxious in the first
   year after their diagnosis. One out of four women who take tamoxifen also
   take an SSRI.

B. Analyzing the excerpt

1. Initial thoughts

What are some of your initial thoughts on this excerpt?
- *The excerpt has high science content.*
- *It uses many long words.*
- *The narrative sometimes gets broken up by parenthetical statements.*
- *The third paragraph contains a very long sentence.*

2. Looking at the *WSEG* score

a. How does this excerpt's average sentence length compare with the
    recommended average of 15 words?

The excerpt has an average sentence length of 23.6 words—more than 1.5 times the recommended average.

b. Count the number of words in each sentence. Then calculate the total number of words for each paragraph. Write your answers in Table 12-1.

Table 12-1. **Words per sentence**

				Sentence				
	1st	*2nd*	*3rd*	*4th*	*5th*	*6th*	*7th*	*Total*
Paragraph 1	10	12	20	22	—	—	—	64
Paragraph 2	36	36	—	—	—	—	—	72
Paragraph 3	21	18	15	11	27	60	20	172
Grand Total								308

c. Is any paragraph longer than 150 words? <u>Yes</u>. If so, do you see a good way to split it into shorter paragraphs?
    The third paragraph is 172 words long. We might consider splitting it into three paragraphs. One could tell why the findings are not surprising. A second could tell how "pharmacoepidemiology is a relative newcomer . . . ." A third could tell why it is hard to study how tamoxifen interacts with SSRIs.

d. For each sentence that uses more than 25 words, do you think it needs to be just one long sentence? Why or why not?
    This excerpt has four sentences longer than 25 words. They could all be broken up into shorter sentences.
    Paragraph 2:
    - *First sentence—We could explain, in one sentence, that Donneyong and colleagues looked at five heath insurance databases. Then, in another sentence, we could tell what information they looked for.*
    - *Second sentence—We could explain, in one sentence, how long their median follow-up was. Then, in another sentence, we could explain their findings.*
    Paragraph 3:
    - *Fifth sentence—We could say that pharmaco-epidemiology is new to the science of drug interactions. Then, in another sentence, we could tell what most studies explored.*
    - *Sixth sentence—We could say, in one sentence, that there are many factors that affect the interaction between tamoxifen and SSRIs that inhibit CYP2D6. Then, in another sentence, we could list them. Then, in yet another sentence, we could tell how these factors work together to attenuate any signal.*

e. Does the reading ease score fall between 45 and 70 (the one standard deviation range)? _No_; or between 33 and 83 (the two standard deviation range)? _No_

f. Does the grade level fall between 6 and 11 (the one standard deviation range)? _No_; or between 4 and 13 (the two standard deviation range)? _No_

3. Looking at grammar

a. For each sentence in the excerpt, underline the <u>subject</u> and double underline the <u>main</u> <u>verb</u>. If the main verb includes a past participle, then draw braces around the {<u>past</u> <u>participle</u>}.

b. Fill in Table 12-2, answering the questions for each sentence.

Table 12-2. **Analyze the grammar of each sentence**

Sentence	*Does the main verb contain a form of* to be?	*Is the sentence active, passive or neither?*	*Is the subject abstract or concrete?*	*Are the subject and verb close together in the first 7–8 words?*
Paragraph 1				
1st	*no*	*active (but sounds like neither)*	*concrete*	*no*
2nd	*yes*	*neither*	*abstract*	*yes*
3rd	*yes*	*neither*	*abstract*	*yes*
4th	*no*	*active*	*abstract*	*yes*
Paragraph 2				
1st	*no*	*active*	*concrete*	*yes*
2nd	*no*	*active*	*concrete*	*no*
Paragraph 3				
1st	*yes*	*neither*	*abstract*	*yes*
2nd	*no*	*active*	*abstract*	*no*
3rd	*no*	*active*	*abstract*	*yes*
4th	*no*	*active*	*abstract*	*yes*
5th	*yes*	*neither*	*abstract*	*yes*
6th	*yes*	*passive*	*concrete*	*no*
7th	*yes*	*neither*	*concrete*	*yes*

c. For each abstract subject, explain, in your own words, why it is abstract.
   - *"One reason/another [reason]" are ideas.*
   - *"Studies/studying/study/it" involve real-world activities guided by abstract thought and analysis.*
   - *"Findings" are ideas.*
   - *"Pharmacoepidemiology" is a field of study.*

d. What words or ideas are written in the plural?

   SSRIs, processes, studies, outcomes, women, results, exceptions, antidepressants, colleagues, databases, years, findings, investigators, inhibitors, interactions, toxicities, drugs, factors, polymorphisms, effects, mechanisms, degrees, reasons, techniques

e. What words or ideas need to be plural?

   SSRIs, processes, studies, outcomes, women, results, colleagues, databases, years, findings, inhibitors, interactions, toxicities, drugs, factors, polymorphisms, effects, degrees, reasons, techniques

f. Fill in Table 12-3 to show your thinking about any phrase that shows possession or connection using *of* or a word ending other than *'s.*

Table 12-3. **Revising phrases that show possession or connection using *of* or a word ending**

List the phrase, underlining *of* or the <u>word ending</u>	Is the possession or connection real world or abstract?	How might you replace *of* or the word ending?
studies <u>of</u> the relation between	*abstract*	*look at the link between*
use <u>of</u> antidepressants	*abstract*	*using anti-depressants*
outset <u>of</u> treatment with tamoxifen	*abstract*	*when they started taking tamoxifen*
median follow-up <u>of</u> about two years	*abstract*	*the median follow up was about two years*
science <u>of</u> drug interactions	*abstract*	*(no change)*
co-prescription <u>of</u> drugs	*abstract*	*when a patient takes two drugs*
degrees <u>of</u> inhibition	*abstract*	*inhibits patients in different degrees*
techniques <u>of</u> pharmacoepidemiology	*abstract*	*(no change)*

4. Prefer the short word

a. Here is a fresh copy of the excerpt. Underline each <u>long word</u>.

> Why does the <u>interaction</u> between <u>tamoxifen</u> and SSRIs remain <u>controversial</u>? One reason is that <u>tamoxifen's</u> <u>pharmacokinetic</u> fate involves processes other than CYP2D6. <u>Another</u> is that studies of the <u>relation</u> between CYP2D6 <u>activity</u> and outcomes in women receiving <u>tamoxifen</u> yield <u>remarkably</u> <u>inconsistent</u> results. <u>Finally</u>, with some <u>exceptions</u>, <u>observational</u> studies show little <u>evidence</u> that use of <u>antidepressants</u> is <u>associated</u> with adverse outcomes in women receiving <u>tamoxifen</u>.
>
> <u>Donneyong</u> and colleagues used data from five US health <u>insurance</u> <u>databases</u> to study women <u>already</u> being treated with an SSRI at the outset of treatment with <u>tamoxifen</u> or who received an SSRI later during its course. Over a <u>median</u> <u>follow-up</u> of about two years, they found no <u>difference</u> in overall <u>mortality</u> among women receiving SSRIs that <u>inhibit</u> CYP2D6 (<u>paroxetine</u> and <u>fluoxetine</u>) <u>relative</u> to SSRIs that do not (<u>citalopram</u>, <u>escitalopram</u>, <u>fluvoxamine</u> and <u>sertraline</u>).
>
> These findings are <u>unsurprising</u>, if for no other reason than <u>follow-up</u> was too brief for any <u>differential</u> <u>survival</u> to show up. Studying total <u>mortality</u> rather than cancer <u>specific</u> outcomes further <u>diminished</u> the <u>investigators'</u> <u>ability</u> to discern signal from noise. <u>Consequently</u>, this study does little to disprove a <u>meaningful</u> <u>interaction</u> between <u>tamoxifen</u> and CYP2D6 <u>inhibitors</u>. It does, however, <u>illustrate</u> just how challenging such studies can be. <u>Pharmacoepidemiology</u> is a <u>relative</u> <u>newcomer</u> to the science of drug <u>interactions</u>, with most studies exploring short term <u>toxicities</u> after the <u>co-prescription</u> of drugs with well <u>established</u> <u>interactions</u>. In contrast, the <u>interaction</u> between <u>tamoxifen</u> and CYP2D6 <u>inhibiting</u> SSRIs is <u>characterized</u> by an <u>elusive</u> outcome (treatment failure), a long latent <u>period</u>, and many other factors (including <u>non-adherence</u>, <u>therapeutic</u> switching, CYP2D6 <u>polymorphisms</u>, <u>dose-response</u> effects, <u>variable</u> <u>mechanisms</u> and degrees of <u>inhibition</u>, and a <u>probable</u> <u>endoxifen</u> threshold below which treatment failure is more likely) that <u>collectively</u> <u>attenuate</u> any signal that might exist. For these reasons, the <u>tamoxifen-SSRI</u> <u>interaction</u> is perhaps the most <u>difficult</u> drug <u>interaction</u> to explore using the techniques of <u>pharmacoepidemiology</u>.

b. Count the number of <u>long words</u> and compute long words as a percent of total words.
<u>80</u> long words/308 total words = <u>26.0</u>%.

c. Double underline any <u>long word</u> you consider a <u>proper</u> <u>name</u> or <u>essential</u> <u>scientific</u> <u>term</u>.

d. For each <u>long word</u> you underlined just once (i.e., skip the essential scientific terms), fill in Table 12-4.

Table 12-4. **Finding shorter words**

Long word	Real world or abstract?	Shorter words that mean about the same thing
interaction	real world	interact, relationship, work together, relate, mix with
controversial	abstract	an issue, uncertain, at question, unsure, discussed
pharmacokinetic	real world	metabolize, metabolism, process, action, working
another	abstract	also, else, more, other, second (reason)
relation/relative	abstract	relate, compare, tie, connect, link
activity	abstract	action, act, active
remarkably	abstract	highly, very, great, notable, remark
inconsistent	abstract	not reliable, changing, irregular, erratic, variable, unable to predict, mixed
finally	abstract	last, third (reason), lastly, also, final
exceptions	abstract	except, a few weren't, omit, odd, not
evidence	real world	data, proof, sign, fact
associated	abstract	related, connected, linked, paired, causes
insurance	abstract	insure
databases	abstract	sources, records, data, info, files
already	abstract	current, now, at that time, being
follow-up	real world	follow up, next, later, after
difference	abstract	differ, gap, not same, change, unlike, not like, reduce
mortality	abstract	death, death rate, number of deaths, mortal
inhibit/-ing/-ors	abstract	prevent, stop, slow, slow down, block

Long word	Real world or abstract?	Shorter words that mean about the same thing
unsurprising	abstract	not surprising, obvious, expected
differential	abstract	differ, difference, favor one
survival	abstract	survive, live, not die, death rate
specific	abstract	unique, only, just for
diminished	abstract	reduce, made small, ebb, shrink, prevent, lower
investigators	real world	researcher
ability	abstract	able, how well they could, strength, effort, skill, can, could, power
consequently	abstract	as a result, therefore, so, then, hence, for that reason, thus
meaningful	abstract	useful, big, key, major
illustrate	abstract	show, prove, point out
newcomer	abstract	new, novice
toxicities	real world	toxin, toxic, poison, poisonous
co-prescription	abstract	prescribed together, prescribe two drugs, give/take two drugs, drugs taken together
established	abstract	known, proven, aware
characterized	abstract	defined, factor, reason
elusive	abstract	to elude, hard to get a good result
period	real world	time, span, phase, stage, delay
non-adherence	abstract	not following doctor's orders, not taking drugs as prescribed, not obeying, not doing
therapeutic	abstract	therapy, treatment, treat, treating
polymorphisms	abstract	different gene form, varying gene form, form of a gene
dose-response	abstract	respond to a dose
variable	abstract	vary, changing, different
mechanisms	abstract	how, how it works, cause and effect
inhibition	abstract	inhibit, prevent, stop, slow down

Long word	Real world or abstract?	Shorter words that mean about the same thing
probable	abstract	likely, may
collectively	abstract	all, all together, taken together, as a whole
attenuate	abstract	mute, make weaker, draw out, indirect, less connected
tamoxifen-SSRI (interaction)	real world	the way tamoxifen interacts with an SSRI
difficult	abstract	hard, complex, not easy

e. Look at the long words listed in Table 12-4. Do any of them have the same or a similar meaning?
- *Mortality and survival*
- *Unsurprising and probable*
- *Diminished and attenuate*

f. Fill in Table 12-5 by listing each long word that is a nominalization and giving the root verb or adjective.

Table 12-5. **Find the root verb or adjective for each nominalization**

Nominalization	Root verb or adjective
interaction	to interact
relation	to relate
activity	to act, active
exceptions	to except
insurance	to insure
follow-up	to follow up
difference	to differ
mortality	mortal
inhibitors	to inhibit
survival	to survive
investigators	to investigate
ability	able
newcomer	to come, new

Nominalization	Root verb or adjective
toxicity	*toxic*
co-prescription	*to prescribe*
non-adherence	*to (not) adhere*
dose-response	*to respond, to dose*
inhibition	*to inhibit*

g. Does the excerpt use any compound word(s) whose meaning or pronunciation might be clearer if hyphenated or written as an open compound? If so, tell which one(s) and why you think so.
    We might hyphenate "pharmaco-kinetic," "pharmaco-epidemiology," and "anti-depressants" so people can better see the two parts.

5. Looking at meaning and logic

a. What is the issue or problem this excerpt deals with?
    Why does the interaction between tamoxifen and SSRIs remain controversial?
b. With regard to this issue or problem, does the excerpt: describe it? tell why it is important? offer a solution?
    It states the question and then answers it.
c. Does the excerpt frame the issue or problem in real-world terms or abstract terms? Or does it only imply the issue or problem?
    The interaction between tamoxifen and an SSRI takes place in the real world— but at a microscopic level within the human body. The excerpt frames the problem of studying this interaction in abstract terms.

C. Prescription for revising

Write your prescription for revising to treat the symptoms of *medicus incomprehensibilis*. List the things you would recommend to help improve reading ease and clarity.
*   *Keep sentence length 15 words average, 25 words maximum*
*   *Introduce and develop one idea in each paragraph*
*   *Revise abstract into concrete*
*   *Observe the 1066 principle*
*   *Avoid using a high percentage of long words*
*   *Keep essential scientific terms; minimize other long words*
*   *Start by anchoring your discussion in the real world*

D. Revision

Revise the excerpt to improve reading ease and clarity.

Why is there still an issue about how <u>tamoxifen</u> *and SSRIs* <u>interact</u>? *One reason is that* <u>tamoxifen</u> <u>metabolism</u> *involves many other factors besides how CYP2D6 acts. A second reason is that those studies that look at the link between the action of CYP2D6 and outcomes in women who take* <u>tamoxifen</u> *have shown mixed results. A third is that only a few studies show any proof that using an* <u>anti-depressant</u> *causes an adverse outcome in a woman who takes* <u>tamoxifen</u>.

<u>Donneyong</u> *et al. studied women who were being treated with an SSRI when they started taking* <u>tamoxifen</u>, *or who started taking an SSRI later during its course. The study used data from five US health* <u>insurance</u> <u>databases</u>. *The* <u>median</u> <u>follow-up</u> *was about two years. During this time, they found no* <u>difference</u> *in* <u>overall</u> *death rate among women taking SSRIs that* <u>inhibit</u> *CYP2D6 (*<u>paroxetine</u> *and* <u>fluoxetine</u>*) and those that don't (*<u>citalopram</u>, <u>escitalopram</u>, <u>fluvoxamine</u> *and* <u>sertraline</u>*).*

These findings are not surprising. The <u>follow-up</u> *was too short for any* <u>difference</u> *in death rate to show up. Studying total death rate rather than cancer* <u>specific</u> *outcomes further reduces the* <u>ability</u> *to discern signal from noise. As a result, this study did little to prove that* <u>tamoxifen</u> *and CYP2D6* <u>inhibitors</u> *do not* <u>interact</u>.

On the other hand, it does show just how hard such studies can be. <u>Pharmaco-epidemiology</u>, *the study of the use and effect of drugs in a* <u>well-defined</u> <u>population</u>, *is a new field. Its methods are new to the science of how drugs* <u>interact</u>. *Most studies look at what happens in the short term when a patient takes two drugs that are known to* <u>interact</u>.

In contrast, there are many factors that make it hard to study how <u>tamoxifen</u> <u>interacts</u> *with an SSRI that* <u>inhibits</u> *CYP2D6. 1. The treatment may fail. 2. There may be a long latent period. 3. The patient may not take the drugs as prescribed. 4. The doctor may switch the treatment. 5.* <u>Different</u> *patients may have* <u>different</u> *forms of the CYP2D6 gene. 6. Not every patient has the same response to the same dose of a drug. 7.* <u>Different</u> *drugs work in* <u>different</u> *ways. 8. The same drug may* <u>inhibit</u> *CYP2D6 in two patients in differing degrees. 9. There may also be an* <u>endoxifen</u> *threshold below which a treatment is more likely to fail. All these factors tend to mute any signal that might exist. For these reasons, the way* <u>tamoxifen</u> <u>interacts</u> *with an SSRI may be hard to explore using the methods of* <u>pharmaco-epidemiology</u>.*

1. Looking at *WSEG* scores

Compute the *WSEG* score for your revision. Fill in Table 12-6 to show how your revision compares with the original.

Table 12-6. **Comparing *WSEG* scores**

WSEG		*Original*	*Revised*	*Change*
W	Number of words	308	416	108
S	Average sentence length	23.6	14.8	−8.8
E	Flesch Reading Ease score	10.8	59.3	48.5
G	Flesch-Kincaid Grade Level	17.6	8.6	−9.0

2. Looking at grammar

Answer the following questions about your revision:

a. Does each sentence put the subject and verb close together within the first 7 or 8 words? If not, tell why it seemed best to do otherwise.
   - *In paragraph 3, third sentence, the subject, "studying," and the verb, "reduces," are separated by an explanation of what they are studying.*
   - *In paragraph 4, second sentence, the subject, "pharmaco-epidemiology," and the verb, "is," are separated by the definition of pharmaco-epidemiology.*

b. Does each sentence use active voice? If not, tell why it seemed best to do otherwise.
   Several sentences are neither active nor passive, since they describe a state of being (e.g., the first sentence). This helps keep the logic of the original.

c. Does each sentence use a concrete subject? If not, tell why it seemed best to use an abstract subject.
   We used several abstract subjects: for example, reason, study, findings, follow-up, pharmaco-epidemiology. This seems appropriate since the excerpt deals with conclusions based on analyzing data.

3. Prefer the short word

a. Underline each long word. Count the number of long words and compute long words as a percent of total words. *46* long words/*416* total words = *11.1*%. Compare your answer with the percent of long words in the original. (See §B.4.b.)

b. Double underline any long word you consider a proper name or essential scientific term.

4. Additional comments

Why did our revision use 108 more words than the original?

The increase resulted from many choices. Here are a few that seemed most significant:
- *We added the definition of pharmacoepidemiology.*
- *The original used a 60-word sentence in paragraph 3, which listed reasons why it is hard to study how tamoxifen and SSRIs interact. We replaced this long sentence with a paragraph that had a topic sentence and listed each reason in its own sentence.*
- *The original also used many long, abstract-sounding terms. But, the way tamoxifen and an SSRI interact inside the human body is something that happens in the real world (even if we can't see it with the naked eye). In light of this, we paraphrased to use shorter words or phrases that sound more concrete.*

Note

1. Quoted in Goodreads, "Justice Louise Brandeis Quotes," https://www.goodreads.com/author/quotes/13738883.Justice_Louis_Brandeis (accessed January 18, 2018).

CHAPTER 13

Analyzing the *WSEG* Scores—What Can We Learn from the Numbers?

The benefits of Plain English are huge—less writing time, shorter documents, higher reader satisfaction. —Plain English Foundation (Australia)[1]

In this book, you examined 12 medical journal excerpts, looking for classic symptoms of *medicus incomprehensibilis*. You assessed those symptoms *subjectively*, using your medical experience and intuition, and *objectively*, by counting and measuring certain things (*percent of long words*, WSEG scores, etc.). You revised to treat the symptoms of *medicus incomprehensibilis*. Your goal was to improve reading ease and clarity, while keeping essential scientific content. You followed up by checking your revision to see how well the treatment reduced the symptoms. We did the same.

All this counting and measuring generated many numbers. In this chapter, we summarize the numbers and consider what we can learn from them.

Percent of long words

Keeping long words under control helps reduce *medicus incomprehensibilis*. Table 13-1 summarizes the percent of long words for the original excerpts and our revisions. Please fill in the information for your revisions.

Table 13-1. **Percent of long words**

Case study	Original excerpt	Our revision	Your revision
1	21.4	8.5	
2	28.0	9.5	
3	17.1	6.1	
4	22.0	11.4	
5	25.5	11.6	

Case study	Original excerpt	Our revision	Your revision
6	28.3	19.1	
7	33.9	11.1	
8	22.6	5.9	
9	24.6	12.3	
10	18.7	8.4	
11	29.4	6.9	
12	26.0	11.1	

This table shows that most original excerpts use 20% to 30% long words. All use more than 17%. By contrast, each of our revisions reduces long words by a wide margin. Most of our revisions use less than 12.5% long words. All use less than 20%.

Figure 13-1 shows the distribution of the percent of long words for the original excerpts and our revisions. It also gives the high, low, mean and median values. Please complete Figure 13-1 by: (1) adding bars to show the distribution of your revisions, and (2) filling in your high, low, mean and median values.

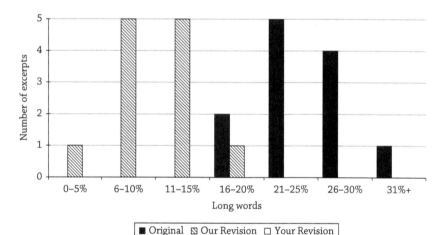

	High	Low	Mean	Median
Originals	33.9	17.1	24.8	25.1
Our revisions	19.1	5.3	10.2	10.3
Your revisions				

Figure 13-1. Distribution of percent of long words

Figure 13-1 shows there is a wide range in the *percent of long words*, both in the originals and our revisions. To a certain extent, this reflects differences in science content. Our revisions reduced the percent of long words a lot. Most original excerpts use more than 20% long words; all use more than 16%. By contrast, most of our revisions use less than 15% long words; all use less than 20%.

WSEG scores

Table 13-2 summarizes the WSEG scores for the original excerpts and our revisions. In the case studies, we gave reading ease scores as our spell-checker does, with any negative score truncated to 0.0. For this analysis, we use negative reading ease scores to get a better mean and range.[2] The table shows how many of the reading ease and grade level scores fall in the recommended one and two standard deviation (s.d.) ranges.[3] Please fill in the table based on your data.

Table 13-2. **Summary of WSEG scores**

| Case study | Original excerpt | | | | Our revision | | | | Your revision | | | |
	W	S	E	G	W	S	E	G	W	S	E	G
1	56	56.0	–1.0	27.3	47	15.6	64.9	8.0				
2	75	25.0	–3.5	19.9	74	14.8	62.6	8.2				
3	82	27.3	12.9	18.2	115	14.3	59.8	8.4				
4	109	21.8	29.4	14.5	114	14.2	65.4	7.6				
5	110	36.6	–1.1	22.5	129	16.1	58.6	9.0				
6	152	38.0	–8.1	23.8	131	18.7	35.4	12.9				
7	180	30.0	–18.9	23.3	234	16.2	55.3	9.5				
8	186	23.2	19.4	16.3	188	14.4	62.1	8.1				
9	207	29.5	16.6	18.2	220	15.7	55.9	9.3				
10	252	126.0	–93.1	57.5	335	13.3	64.3	7.6				
11	272	34.0	10.0	19.3	262	17.4	63.4	8.7				
12	308	23.6	10.8	17.6	416	14.8	59.3	8.6				
1 s.d. range	—	—	0	0	—	—	11	11	—	—		
2 s.d. range	—	—	0	0	—	—	12	12	—	—		

Now, let's take a closer look at each item of WSEG.

Number of words *(W)*

If we compare the number of words for the original excerpts and our revisions, we see that four of our revisions use fewer words (CS 1, 2, 6 and 11). Four use a few more words (CS 4, 5, 8 and 9). Together, these eight revisions use a few less words than the original excerpts.

The striking difference comes with our revisions for CS 3, 7, 10 and 12, where our revisions use 30–40% more words. For these revisions, we added many more words as we tried to improve the flow of logical reasoning. (See the comments at the end of our answers for these case studies.)

Figure 13-2 compares the number of words for the original excerpts and our revisions and gives the high, low, mean and median values. Please add bars to show the number of words for your revisions, and fill in the high, low, mean and median values.

This figure shows that the overall increase in words relates solely to the four revisions where we try to improve logical reasoning.

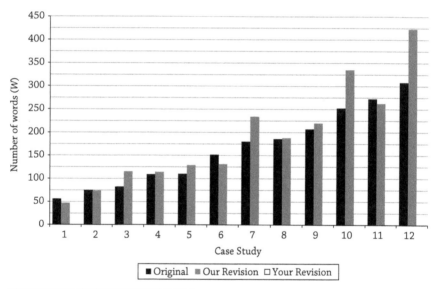

	High	Low	Mean	Median
Originals	308	56	166	166
Our revisions	416	47	189	159.5
Your revisions				

Figure 13-2. Number of words *(W)*

Average sentence length (s)

Keeping sentence length under control also helps reduce *medicus incomprehensibilis*. Table 13-2 shows that the original excerpts tend to use long sentences. Their average sentence lengths range widely, from 21.8 to 126.0 words.

By contrast, our revisions use shorter sentences. The average sentence lengths range more narrowly, from 13.3 to 18.7 words.

Figure 13-3 shows the distribution of average sentence lengths for the original excerpts and our revisions. It also gives the high, low, mean and median values. Please add bars to show the distribution of your revisions, and fill in your high, low, mean and median values.

Figure 13-3 shows that the original excerpts use long sentences. Their average sentence lengths range widely. The mean *average sentence length* for all originals is 39.3; the median is 29.8.

By contrast, our revisions use shorter sentences, with a narrower range of average sentence lengths. The mean *average sentence length* for all our revisions is 15.5; the median, 15.2.

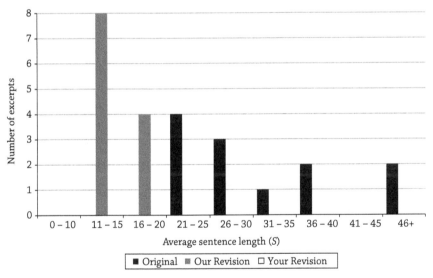

	High	*Low*	*Mean*	*Median*
Originals	21.8	126.0	39.3	29.8
Our revisions	13.3	18.7	15.5	15.2
Your revisions				

Figure 13-3. Distribution of average sentence length (S)

Flesch Reading Ease score (*E*)

Table 13-2 shows that the reading ease scores for the original excerpts are low and range widely (from –93.1 to 29.4). None of the reading ease scores for the original excerpts falls in the one or two standard deviation ranges.

By contrast, our revisions achieve much higher reading ease scores, and those scores range in a narrower band (from 35.4 to 65.4). The reading ease scores for most of our revisions fall in the one standard deviation range. All fall in the two standard deviation range.

Figure 13-4 shows the distribution of reading ease scores for the original excerpts and our revisions. It also gives the high, low, mean and median values. Please add bars to show the distribution of reading ease scores for your revisions, and fill in your high, low, mean and median values.

Figure 13-4 shows that all of the original excerpts have low reading ease scores, and these scores vary widely. The mean reading ease score for all originals is –2.2, the median, 4.5.

By contrast, our revisions have much higher reading ease scores, and these scores vary in a narrower range. The mean reading ease score for our revisions is 58.9; the median, 61.0.

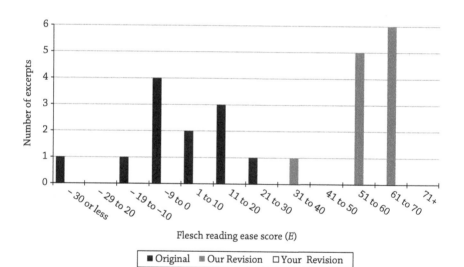

Flesch reading ease score (*E*)

■ Original   ■ Our Revision   □ Your Revision

	High	Low	Mean	Median
Originals	29.4	–93.1	–2.2	4.5
Our revisions	65.4	35.4	58.9	61.0
Your revisions				

Figure 13-4. Distribution of reading ease scores (*E*)

Flesch-Kincaid Grade Level (*G*)

Table 13-2 shows that the grade levels for the original excerpts are high and range widely, from 14.5 to 57.5. None of the grade levels for the original excerpts falls in the one or two standard deviation range. The grade levels for our revisions are much lower and range more narrowly, from 7.6 to 12.9. The grade levels for most of our revisions fall in the one standard deviation range; all fall in the two standard deviation range.

Figure 13-5 shows the distribution of grade levels for the original excerpts and our revisions. It also gives the high, low, mean and median values. Please add bars to show the distribution of grade levels for your revisions, and fill in your high, low, mean and median values.

Figure 13-5 shows how the original excerpts tend to have high grade levels, and those grade levels range widely. The mean grade level for the original excerpts is 23.2; the median, 19.6.

By contrast, most of our revisions have grade levels from 7 to 9. Only one has a grade level from 10 to 12. The mean grade level for our revisions is 8.8; the median, 8.5.

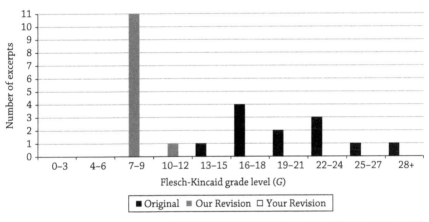

	High	Low	Mean	Median
Originals	57.5	14.5	23.2	19.6
Our revisions	12.9	7.6	8.8	8.5
Your revisions				

Figure 13-5. Distribution of grade level scores (*G*)

Summary

This chapter analyzed the WSEG scores for the case studies. These scores show that our revisions drastically reduced the symptoms of *medicus incomprehensibilis* in every case. We hope you can say the same.

Notes

1. Plain English Foundation (Australia), "Home page," https://www.plainenglishfoundation. com/home (accessed February 6, 2018).
2. We computed negative reading ease scores using the Flesch Reading Ease and Flesch-Kincaid Grade Level formulas; Wikipedia, s.v. "Flesch–Kincaid readability tests" https:// en.wikipedia.org/wiki/Flesch–Kincaid_readability_tests (accessed December 4, 2017); the WSEG score gave us the data we needed to compute the reading ease score, except for total number of syllables. We found the total number of syllables by using the grade level formula and solving for the number of syllables.
3. For a reminder of what these ranges are, see Table I-1 in the Introduction.

CHAPTER 14

Afterword

Simple can be harder than complex: You have to work hard to get your thinking clean to make it simple. But it's worth it in the end because, once you get there, you can move mountains. —Steve Jobs[1]

In these case studies, we looked at 12 medical journal excerpts that showed classic symptoms of *medicus incomprehensibilis*. Each one provided a real-world medical writing situation for you to practice on. Together, they use about 2,000 words—less than the length of one medical journal article.

In each case study, you reviewed, analyzed and revised one excerpt. You tried to keep essential scientific content, while improving reading ease and clarity. By now, you know this isn't always easy, but the results are worth it.

These case studies helped you practice using some new revising strategies. We hope this book provided the extra practice you needed to master the tips from *Plain English for Doctors*, so you can apply them to your own writing.

Note

1. Interview with *Business Week*, 1998, quoted in *BBC News*, "In Quotes: Apple's Steve Jobs," October 6, 2011. http://www.bbc.com/news/world-us-canada-15195448 (accessed February 5, 2018).

GLOSSARY

The 1066 Principle the general tendency for English speakers to use short words to talk about the real world, and long words, more sparingly, to talk about abstract ideas.

Abstract a theoretical way of looking at things; something that exists only in idealized form. A term is abstract if it relates to the world of ideas, including a concept, theory, calculation or procedure. Contrast with *concrete*.

Active voice A sentence is in active voice when its subject is *doing* the action. See *voice*.

Clear Writing is *"clear"* when the narrative uses words and concepts familiar to the reader. Ideally, a reader can understand and vividly imagine the article on first reading without having to *study* it. The reader remembers each key idea.

Closed compound a compound word written as one word (e.g., *multicell, hyperadrenergic, vaso-motor,* and *sinoatrial*). See *compound word*.

Compound word or ***compound*** a word formed by combining two or more words, or a word plus a prefix. The three main types of compounds are the *open compound* (e.g., *student nurse*), the *closed compound* (e.g., *multicell*), and the *hyphenated compound* (e.g., *pre-menstrual*).

Concise Writing is *"concise"* when it demands as little of the reader's mental energy as possible. This usually means short while still clear. Good writing involves tradeoffs. A few short words may convey the message more vividly than one long, but lifeless word. Writing concisely often means cutting any unnecessary word; but sometimes, cutting too many words makes the message cryptic and harder to understand.

Concrete something from the real world (e.g., a doctor, a patient, a bed, a test tube). Contrast with *abstract*.

Elegant variation varying terms to make writing more interesting. Technical writing tends to avoid elegant variation, but it is common in other types of writing.

Essential scientific content important scientific ideas an author must include in their article.

Essential scientific term a long word that helps convey essential scientific content clearly and concisely. An essential scientific term meets four tests:

1. No shorter word serves just as well,
2. You can't paraphrase in a few short words,
3. Doctors and other medical scientists use the term consistently (i.e., exclusively), and
4. It's easy to look up in a standard reference.

Flesch Reading Ease a readability test that indicates how difficult it is to read a passage in English. The scores generally range from 0.0 to 100.0.

Flesch-Kincaid Grade Level a readability test that assigns a USA school grade level or year to a passage in English.

Hyphenated compound a compound word where words are written together but separated by a hyphen (e.g., *pre-menstrual, cost-effective, one-time, self-reported*). See *compound word*.

Insider somebody who knows the science and vocabulary of a particular specialized field. *Insiders* are the narrowest possible definition of the potential audience for an article. Contrast with the *widest reasonable audience*.

Long word any word with three or more syllables, but not including a two-syllable word that becomes a three-syllable word by adding a common ending, such as *-ed, -es* or *-ing*.

Medicus incomprehensibilis a condition that affects doctors and other medical scientists and causes them to write dull, lifeless prose that is hard to understand. *Medicus incomprehensibilis* is primarily caused by needless grammatical complexity.

Narrative pathway the direction of a narrative, or a conceptual program for organizing a narrative.

Nominalization the process of making an abstract noun out of a verb or adjective.

Open compound a compound word, where words work together, but are written as separate words (e.g., *student nurse, 50 percent, reference book*). See *compound word*.

Passive voice A sentence is in passive voice when its subject receives the action. See *voice*.

Past participle a form of the verb that expresses completed action.[1] A past participle is usually the same form as the verb in past tense. For regular verbs, this means adding a *-d* or *-ed* ending (e.g., *worked, decided, starved*). Irregular verbs use irregular forms (e.g., *broken, swum*).[2] Examples:

- "The results of the meta-analysis of treatment effect of lubiprostone vs. placebo are shown in Figures 2 and 3."[3] In this sentence, *shown* is a past participle.
- "It may be specified in the protocol of a prospective accuracy study, for instance, that to reduce study costs or burden to patients only a randomly selected subset of patients in a specific subgroup are to be verified by the preferred reference standard."[4] In this sentence, *specified, selected, verified*, and *preferred* are past participles.

Plain English writing that conveys the right content, clearly and concisely. Writing in plain English involves sharpening up the medical science to make it clearer and more accessible to the widest reasonable audience.

Short word a one- or two-syllable word. This also includes a two-syllable word that becomes a three-syllable word by adding a common ending, such as *-ed, -es*, or *-ing*. Contrast with *long word*.

Shorter word a word that has fewer syllables.

Subject (grammar) the noun or pronoun that agrees with the verb.[5] A noun functioning as a subject is the actor, person, or thing about which an assertion is made in a clause.[6] Examples:

- "Onychomycosis is a fungal infection of the nails that causes discoloration, thickening, and separation from the nail bed."[7] In this sentence, *Onychomycosis* is the subject.
- "Identification of hyphae, pseudohyphae, or spores confirms infection but does not identify the organism."[8] Here, *Identification* is the subject. (The phrase, *"Identification of hyphae, pseudohyphae, or spores,"* is the *logical* subject.[9])

Verb expresses an action, occurrence or a state of being.[10] Examples:

- "Diagnostic studies typically <u>evaluate</u> the accuracy of one or more tests, markers, or models by comparing their results with those of, ideally, a 'gold' reference test or standard."[11] Here, the verb is *evaluate*.
- "High K⁺ intake also <u>has</u> a stimulatory effect on the release of aldosterone at the level of the adrenal gland."[12] Here, the verb is *has*.

Vivid language language that is clear, detailed, powerful, full of life, and strikingly alive.

Voice a term that describes whether the subject of the sentence is doing or receiving the action. See *active voice; passive voice*.

Widest reasonable audience the widest reasonable audience for a journal article includes anybody with an interest in the science, whether or not they are an *insider* in the field. It includes a doctor or scientist working in the same specialty, another specialty, or even another discipline. It includes someone living or educated in an English-speaking country or elsewhere, whether they are a native speaker of English or not. It includes readers at different levels of training. It includes a regular journal subscriber and somebody who searches for an article on the Internet. Contrast with *insider*.

WSEG four items of data helpful for assessing reading ease for a writing sample: the number of <u>w</u>ords (*W*), average <u>s</u>entence length (*S*), Flesch Reading <u>E</u>ase score (*E*), and Flesch-Kincaid <u>G</u>rade Level (*G*). We write a *WSEG score* for a writing sample in the form (*WSEG = 55/55.0/0.2/26.8*).

Notes

1. *Chicago Manual of Style*, 15th ed. (Chicago: University of Chicago Press, 2003), sec. 5.103.
2. Joseph Williams, *Style: Lessons in Clarity and Grace*, 9th ed. (New York: Pearson, Longman, 2007), 266.
3. Fan Li et al., "Lubiprostone Is Effective in the Treatment of Chronic Idiopathic Constipation and Irritable Bowel Syndrome: A Systematic Review and Meta-Analysis of Randomized Controlled Trials," *Mayo Clin Proc* 91, no. 4, (2016): 461.
4. Christiana Naaktgeboren et al., "Anticipating Missing Reference Standard Data When Planning Diagnostic Accuracy Studies," *BMJ* 352 (2016), under "The problem: missing reference standard data," https://www.bmj.com/content/352/bmj.i402.
5. Martin Cutts, *Oxford Guide to Plain English*, 3rd ed. (Oxford, UK: Oxford University Press, 2009), 122.
6. *Chicago Manual of Style*, 15th ed. (Chicago: University of Chicago Press, 2003), sec 5.23.
7. Dyanne P. Westerberg and Michael J. Voyack, "Onychomycosis: Current Trends in Diagnosis and Treatment," *Am Fam Phys* 88, no. 11 (2013), 762.
8. Ibid., 762.
9. See Joseph Williams, *Style: Lessons in Clarity and Grace*, 9th ed. (New York: Pearson Longman, 2007), 81–82.
10. *Merriam-Webster's Learner's Dictionary*, Merriam-Webster.com, s.v. "Verb," https://www.merriam-webster.com/dictionary/verb (accessed July 11, 2016).
11. Christiana Naaktgeboren et al., "Anticipating Missing Reference Standard Data When Planning Diagnostic Accuracy Studies," *BMJ* 352, no. 8044 (2016), under "The problem: missing reference standard data," https://www.bmj.com/content/352/bmj.i402.
12. Biff F. Palmer and Deborah J. Clegg, "Achieving the Benefits of High-Potassium Paleolithic Diet, without the Toxicity," *Mayo Clin Proc* 91, no. 4 (2016): 500.

RESOURCES

Books

Cutts, Martin. *Oxford Guide to Plain English*. Oxford: Oxford University Press, 2009.

Greene, Anne E. *Writing Science in Plain English*. Chicago: University of Chicago Press, 2013.

Iverson, Cheryl, et al. *AMA Manual of Style*. 10th ed. Oxford, UK: Oxford University Press, 2007.

Linares, Oscar, David Daly and Gertrude Daly. *Plain English for Doctors and Other Medical Scientists*, New York: Oxford University Press, 2017.

Stedman's Medical Dictionary. 28th ed. Philadelphia: Lippincott Williams & Wilkins, 2006.

Williams, Joseph M., and Joseph Bizup. *Style: Lessons in Clarity and Grace*. 11th ed. New York: Pearson, 2015.

Internet

Centers for Disease Control and Prevention. "Plain Language Materials and Resources." https://www.cdc.gov/healthliteracy/developmaterials/plainlanguage.html.

National Institutes of Health. "Plain Language at NIH." https://www.nih.gov/institutes-nih/nih-office-director/office-communications-public-liaison/clear-communication/plain-language.

Plain Language Action and Information Network. *Federal Plain Language Guidelines* (March 2011, revised May 2011). http://www.plainlanguage.gov/howto/guidelines/FederalPLGuidelines/FederalPLGuidelines.pdf.

Plain Language Campaign. "Writing Medical Information in Plain English." http://www.plainenglish.co.uk/files/medicalguide.pdf

The Royal Children's Hospital of Melbourne. "Guide to Writing in Plain Language." http://www.rch.org.au/uploadedFiles/Main/Content/ethics/Writing%20Tips.pdf.

INDEX

References to figures and tables are denoted by an italicized *f* and *t*.